# INTEGRATING CHINESE AND WESTERN MEDICINE
## A HANDBOOK
## FOR PRACTITIONERS

Zhang Junwen    Bai Yongquan
Chen Longshun

FOREIGN LANGUAGES PRESS    BEIJING

First Edition 1993

ISBN 0-8351-2845-8
ISBN 7-119-01492-7

© Foreign Languages Press, Beijing, 1993

Published by Foreign Languages Press
24 Baiwanzhuang Road, Beijing 100037, China

Printed by Beijing Foreign Languages Printing House
19 Chegongzhuang Xilu, Beijing 100044, China

Distributed by China International Book Trading Corporation
35 Chegongzhuang Xilu, Beijing 100044, China
P.O. Box 399, Beijing, China

*Printed in the People's Republic of China*

# Contents

# Foreword

This book is intended to provide effective management of certain common illnesses with combined therapies of traditional Chinese medicine and Western medicine, each having its own advantages that the other does not have. In the past three decades, we have experimented and researched trying to combine these two different medicines together by taking from each the most effective approaches. In our research, we have found that many illnesses can be better or completely cured with combined therapies than with any methods of either of the two medicines alone. Certain illnesses, which can not be satisfactorily dealt with using Western medicine, can be effectively cured using traditional Chinese medicine, and vice versa. Or some illnesses, which have no effective management in either Western medicine or traditional Chinese medicine, can be perfectly managed with the combined therapies.

The book discusses the treatment of 43 diseases in its 14 chapters, most of which have been used as parts of a medical textbook for our students and students from other countries who came to learn traditional Chinese medicine in our university. The combined therapies described in the book are so widely practised in our hospitals that they have become a new medicine based on both Western medicine and traditional Chinese medicine.

We are very glad to be able to say that in preparing this book we have had the assistance of many doctors in our university. We are grateful to them for their suggestions, review and permission to use their materials in this book.

The Authors
Xi'an Medical University
Xi'an, Shaanxi

# *Preface*

Traditional Chinese and Western medicines are the two kinds of medicines that had been developed in different historical environments in man's struggle against illnesses, but due to various historical reasons and limits, each has its own advantages and disadvantages that the other does not have. Traditional Chinese medicine is characterized by the concept of wholism which views the various parts of the human body as an organic whole emphasizing the harmony and coordination of the internal organs with other parts or structures and the unity of the human body with the external environment; as well as by the theory for diagnosis and treatment based on overall analysis of symptoms and signs, the cause, nature and location of the illness and the physical condition of the patient. Western medicine is closely related with modern knowledge of science and technology, providing better skills and equipment for examination, diagnosis and treatment of certain illnesses. Combined Western and traditional Chinese medicine is a new medicine that combines the above advantages of the two schools of medicine.

Through the joint efforts of the doctors of both schools in researches and experiments in the past few decades, a new medicine has been established with new theories and various effective therapies that surpass those from which they have been created and can effectively solve a lot of health problems that cannot be cured or relieved with Western or traditional Chinese medicine alone. And for this reason, to study traditional Chinese medicine, particularly acupuncture and herbs, has been the rage in the world today.

The authors of this book have been engaged in clinical research and practice on combined management in a well-equipped university hospital for over thirty years. Their efforts are a dedication both to medical science and to the health of human beings. Their book summarizes the valuable achievements and experiences of their work and describes in a well-organized setting the valuable managements that have been proved effective in the researches and are being widely practiced in patient care in China. I believe that the book will be a good companion for all doctors at home and abroad.

**Zhang Baozhen, M.D.**
Xi'an, Shaanxi Province

# Chapter I
# DISEASES OF THE RESPIRATORY SYSTEM

## 1. ACUTE UPPER RESPIRATORY TRACT INFECTION

### GENERAL CONSIDERATION

Infection of the respiratory tract is perhaps one of the most common human ailments and is a source of discomfort, disability and loss of time for most average adults. It is also a substantial cause of morbidity and serious illnesses in young children and in the elderly, including inflammation of nasal tract, nasopharynx, pharynx and larynx. Most cases are caused by virus such as rhinovirus, parainfluenza, respiratory syncytial virus, adenovirus, influenza A, B and C virus, etc., but some by bacteria such as pneumococcus, hemolytic streptococcus, hemophilus and staphylococcus. Many of these viral infections run their natural course in older children and in adults without specific treatment and without great risk of bacterial complications. In young infants and in the elderly, or in persons with impaired respiratory tract function, bacterial superinfection increases morbidity and mortality rates.

In traditional Chinese medicine, this condition is often called seasonal disease or external affection, which refers to the disease or the symptoms caused by the six pathogenic factors, namely wind, cold, summer-heat, dampness, dryness, fire, as well as malignant infections and pathogenic factors.

### CLINICAL MANIFESTATIONS

Acute upper respiratory tract infections generally are divided into the following five types:

Common cold. This familiar syndrome is characterized mainly by nasal obstruction with discharge, sore throat, sneezing, hoarseness, varying degrees of malaise, cough, sinusitis and otitis. Fever is usually absent in adults but may be present in small children.

Croup (Laryngotracheobronchitis). This is most commonly a parainfluenza virus infection of small children with anatomic location in the subglottal area. It produces hoarseness, a "seal bark" cough and signs of upper airway obstruction with inspiratory stridor xiphoid and suprasternal retraction, but no pain on swallowing.

1

Herpangina. This disorder is commonly a coxsackie A virus infection of small children with sore throat and fever. The epiglottis is markedly swollen with a cherry red appearance.

Pharyngo conjunctival fever. The causes of this disorder are adenovirus, coxsackie and influenza A, B and C virus, and it is characterized mainly by fever, sore throat, increased discharge in the eyes, photophobia and congestion of conjunctiva.

Bacterial pharyngotonsillitis. The most common cause of the illness is hemolytic-streptococcus, pneumococcus and staphylococcus. Its features are abrupt onset with chills and fever, and marked congestion of the pharynx. The temperature is above 39°C and the tonsil is enlarged with yellowish exudate on the superficial mucosa.

## DIAGNOSIS

Essentials of diagnosis are:
- Abrupt onset with fever, chills, malaise, cough, coryza and muscle aches.
- Pain, fever and catarrhal symptoms.
- Secondary bacterial infection with increased white blood cell.
- Chest x-ray is normal.

## TREATMENT

Bed rest is important to reduce complications, and analgesics and sedative cough mixture may be used. Antibiotics should be reserved for treatment of bacterial complications. Antihistamines are of value only in allergic or vasomotor rhinitis.

In traditional Chinese medicine, herbal therapy and acupuncture therapy are very effective for this disease, and the disorder is recognized as two different types caused by wind and cold, and wind and heat.

Flu caused by wind and cold shows the chief symptoms such as fever, chills, headache, nasal obstruction and thin nasal discharge. The patient usually does not feel thirsty, but has a superficial and tense pulse. The tongue is found covered with a thin whitish coating. The general rules for the treatment of this type are to use strong sudorific drugs pungent in taste and warming in property to dispel wind and cold in external symptom-complex. The most effective formula is Jin Fang Bai Du San Jia Jian.

Constituents:

Jingjie (herb)  12g
Fangfeng (root)  12g
Chinese thorowax  15-30g
Root of purple-flowered peucedanum  15g
Notopterygium  12g
Angelica (root)  10g
Chuanxiong (rhizome)  12g
Peppermint (herb)  10g

    Apricot kernel  12g
    Tatarian aster  20g
    Common coltsfoot flower  10g
    Licorice root  6g

Decoction and dosage. Put all the above herbs together to be simmered twice, then the broth of each mixed, half of the mixed broth each time, twice a day.

If high fever has continued for two days, 30 grams of gypsum is added to the above formula.

If cough attacks very often, tendril-leaved fritillary bulb (10g) and Pinellia (tuber) (10g) are put on the formula.

If headache is frequent, root of herbaceous peony (12g) and Ligusticum (rhizome) (12g) are increased in the formula.

Flu caused by wind and heat usually manifests fever, headache, perspiration, chilly sensation, thirst and pain of the throat. The pulse is superficial and rapid and the tongue is covered with thin, white or slightly yellowish coating with red edge and tip. The rules for treatment are the same as those for wind and cold type. The effective formula is Yin Xiao San Jia Jian.

    Constituents:

    Honeysuckle flower  15-30g
    Weeping forsythia  15-30g
    Bamboo leaves  10g
    Jingjie (herb)  12g
    Achene of great burdock  10g
    Peppermint (herb)  10g
    Common reed rhizome  30g
    Root of balloonflower  30g
    Root of Zhejiang figwort  15-30g
    Tuber of dwarf lilyturf  18g
    Fresh or dried root of rehmannia  18g
    Gypsum  30g
    Licorice root  6g

Decoction and dosage is the same.

If the patient has high fever, the dose of Gypsum should be doubled and root of Zhejiang figwort (30g) is added.

If the patient complains of sore throat, boat-fruited sterculia (seed) (4 Pieces) is added.

Besides, some herb pills such as Yin Xiao Jian Du Pills, Lin Xiao Jian Du Pills, Jiu Wei Jiang Huo Pills, Qiang Li Yin Xiao Tablet, and Sang Ju Gan Mao Tablet are also the effective herbal drugs.

Acupuncture therapy is proved to be especially effective for this disorder and the prescriptions are:

A. For wind-cold type

Main points: GV16 Fengfu and G20 Fengchi.

Auxiliary points: Taiyang (extra) for headache and Ying Xiang (extra) for nasal obstruction.

B. For wind-heat type

Points: GV14 Dazhui, G20 Fengchi, TE5 Waiguan, LI4 Hegu and L11 Shao-shang.

Method: All the above points are punctured with moderate stimulation and the needles are retained for 30 minutes. One course includes ten punctures.

For the management of upper respiratory tract infection, our experience tells us that herbal drugs are more effective than the chemicals, particularly the decoctions which have a quick and most powerful effect.

## 2. CHRONIC BRONCHITIS

### GENERAL CONSIDERATION

The definition of chronic bronchitis requires that productive cough be present on most days for a minimum of three months in the year in at least two consecutive years in order to make the diagnosis. The disease is probably the most common debilitating respiratory disease in China. There is a strong association with inhalation of irritant substance such as various forms of air pollution and heavy smokers. The pathologic findings include hyperplasia and hypertrophy of the submucosal bronchial mucous glands, hyperplasia of bronchiolar goblet cells, sequamous metaplasia of bronchial mucosal cells, chronic and acute inflammatory infiltrates in the bronchial submucosa, profuse inflammatory exudates in the lumens of brochi and bronchioles and denudation of bronchial mucosa.

In traditional Chinese medicine, this disorder is called "Ke Sou" and is thought to be caused by damp, cold and heat phlegm and deficiency of the lungs.

### CLINICAL MANIFESTATIONS

The hallmark of chronic bronchitis is chronic cough and sputum production. Productive cough may be present on most of the days, at least for many years. The disease is commonly seen in old men and women with an onset related to winter and is caused by cold. At early stage, cough is productive and often occurs in the morning. This may be the only symptoms and may gradually become serious and symptoms such as dyspnea on exertion may develop.

As the disease progresses, the course of the illness is usually marked by recurrent episodes of acute respiratory failure resulting from infectious exacerbations of the bronchitis. Clinically, the manifestations are increased cough, change in sputum from clear and mucoid to purulent, fever, dyspnea and varying degrees of respiratory distress. The course of the disease is one of gradual increase in frequency and severity of episodes of acute infection and respiratory failure, eventually resulting in intubation and the need for almost constant ventilatory assistance. Death usually occurs during an episode of respiratory failure.

The physical findings vary with the stage in which the patient is examined.

During relatively quiescent period, the only findings may be increased anteroposterior diameter of the chest, hyperresonance to percussion, prolonged expiratory phase, scattered diffuse coarse or moderate rhonchi and rales and wheezing. Later the patient may manifest the signs and symptoms of pulmonary hypertension and right ventricular failure, i.e. increased second heart sound, pedal edema, hepatomegaly and ascites.

If examined during an acute attack, the patient is found in respiratory distress as evidenced by tachypnea and use of accessory muscles for respiration. Cough is often prominent and cyanosis during acute attack is not uncommon.

## DIAGNOSIS

Essentials of diagnosis:

• Productive cough be present on most days for a minimum of 3 months in the year in at least two consecutive years.

• During relatively quiescent period, the only finding may be increased anteroposterior diameter of the chest. Other findings such as hyperresonance to percussion, prolonged expiratory phase, scattered diffuse coarse or moderate rhonchi and rales and wheezing are also present.

• Chest x-ray shows  evidence of pulmonary overinflation with increased anteroposterior diameter, flattened diaphragm and increased retrosternal air space. There are often prominent and increased bronchial markings at the lung base as parallel or tapering shadows ("tram lines") which reflect the increased thickness of the bronchial wall.

## TREATMENT

The patient should be vigorously encouraged to discontinue cigrette smoking and avoid exposure to other toxic inhalants and postural drainage exercises when possible. The preferred drug is Ampicillin or Erythromycin and Tab Amnophylline for five to seven days.

In traditional Chinese medicine, this disorder is divided into cold-phlegm and heat-phlegm types, the therapy of each varies.  Cold-phlegm is characterized clinically by cough with copious and easily coughed up sputum and relief of cough after expectoration and accompanied by such symptoms as a feeling of suppression of the chest, poor appetite, white glossy coating of the tongue, superficial and slippery pulse, etc. But the heat type is due to the accumulation and retention of the phlegm and the pathogenic heat in the lungs with major symptoms such as cough, dyspnea, yellowish thin or bloody sputum, chest and hypochondriac pain, red tongue with yellowish glossy coating, smooth and rapid pulse.

*1. Herb therapy*

For chronic bronchitis caused by cold phlegm. The rules of treatment are to dry the dampness and to eliminate phlegm. The formula is Er Chen Tang Jia Jian.

Constituents:

Dried old orange peel   12g

Pinellia (tuber)   12g
Tuckahoe   12-13g
Tatarian aster (root) 15-30g
Common coltsfoot flower  10g
Root of purple-flowered peucedanum   15g
Apricot kernel  12g
Bulb of fritillary   10g
Perillaseed   15g
Root of the narrow-leaved polygala   12g
Licorice root   6g

Decoction and dosage. All the above herbs make a dose and six to ten doses are prescribed with one dose daily. Each dose is simmered twice and then the broth of each mixed, half of the mixed broth each time, twice a day.

For chronic bronchitis caused by heat phlegm. The rules of treatment are to eliminate phlegm and clear pathogenic heat. The formula is Qin Jin Hua Tan Yang Jia Jian.
Constituents:

Skullcap  12g
Capejasmine (fruit)  12g
Root of balloonflower  12g
Tuber of dwarf lilyturf  12-18g
Root-bark of white mulberry  18g
Bulb of fritillary   10g
Rhizome of wind-weed   10g
Seed of Mongolian snakeground 12g
Tangerine peel   12g
Cordate houttuynia   30g

Decoction and dosage is the same.

If there is blood in the sputum, the following herbs are added to the formula: donkey-hide gelatin 10-12g, node of lotus rhizome 12-30g, hyacinth bletilla 15-20g and root of pseudo-ginseng 3g.

*2. Acupuncture therapy*

Points along the Taiyin (lung) and Yang-ming (the large intestine) Channels are selected to activate the dispersing function of the lung and to relieve the phlegm-damp.

Points: L7 Lieque, LI4 Hegu, B13 Feishu and L5 Chize.

Method: All the above points are punctured with moderate stimulation and the needles are retained for 20 to 30 minutes.

*3. Cutting therapy*

Points for cutting: B12 Fengmen and B13 Feishu.

Method: Both of the points are cut and the procedure is seen in Chapter XII.

*4. Plum-blossom needle therapy*

Peck with plum-blossom needle along the Du and Urinary Bladder Channels on the upper part of the back till the skin becomes red or bleeds slightly.

*5. Ear-acupuncture therapy*

Points: Lung Pt and Asthma Pt.

Method: The therapy is given once daily or once every other day. The needles are retained for 30 to 60 minutes and a course includes ten punctures.

In addition, some proprietary herb drugs are also available in China for this disease. Tangerine Peel Pills, Xiao Ke Chun Cough Solution, Xin Su Cough Solution and Pinellia Cough Solution are advisable for cold phlegm type. Er Mu Nin Cough Pills and Chuan Bei Cough Tablets are good for heat phlegm type.

The most effective way to treat chronic bronchitis is the combination of Chinese herbal decoction with antibiotics. Antibiotics are very effective against bacterial and secondary infections while Chinese herbal decoction is good for eliminating the phlegm.

# 3. BRONCHIAL ASTHMA

## GENERAL CONSIDERATION

Asthma is a bronchial hypersensitive disorder characterized by reversible airway obstruction caused by a combination of mucosal edema, constriction of the bronchial musculature and excessive secretion of viscid mucus.

In asthma, there is a continuous state of hyperreactivity of the bronchi, during which exposure to a wide variety of bronchial irritants will precipitate an asthmatic attack.

In normal subjects, inhalation of histamine or carbachol may cause a little increase in airway resistance. By contrast, the bronchi of the patients with asthma are highly reactive and show marked bronchoconstriction in response to these substances. This phenomenon is termed bronchial hyperreactivity. In addition to these pharmacologic agents, bronchial hyperreactivity has also been shown to occur with a variety of nonspecific irritants such as dusts and cold air. In subjects with seasonal grasspollen asthma, hyperreactivity increases during the pollen season whether attacks are occurring or not. In subjects with hyperreactivity associated with nonallergic states, e.g. chronic bronchitis, clinical observation of the effects of removal of inhaled irritants such as smoking or moving to a less polluted environment suggests that some degree of reversibility is possible. A number of factors may cause hyperreactive bronchi to constrict and for convenience they are all termed irritants. Although the end-result of their action is similar, it is important clinically to decide whether the irritant acts by inducing an allergic reaction or by some other mechanism because specific therapy is available only for the allergic type.

This disease is called Xiao Chuan in traditional Chinese medicine, which simply means asthma and is thought to be an illness with the combination of wheezing and dyspnea. Dyspnea is characterized by wheezing sound in the throat with the symptom complex such as rapid shallow breathing and flapping of alae nasi. The mouth of the patient is open and his shoulders become elevated and he is unable to lie flat.

## CLINICAL MANIFESTATIONS

Asthma occurs characteristically as episodes which may last from a few minutes to several days with a wide range of severity. Between attacks the patient is well. Alternatively, the condition may be associated with chronic airflow obstruction and some symptoms may then be present continuously though of varying severity.

In severe attacks, the patient is extremely dyspneic, orthpneic and often cyanosed. He is agitated and may be confused. He is often most comfortable sitting forward with his arms leaning on some support, a point to remember when asking the patient to lean back on the pillows to be examined. There is indrawing of the soft tissues of the neck and the accessory muscles are active. The chest is overinflated with diminished hepatic and cardiac dullness to percussion and respiratory movement is reduced. High pitched sibilant rhonchi which are often associated with coarse crepitations in some areas, occur during inspiration as well as expiration. It is important to remember that when airflow obstruction becomes extreme, rhonchi may disappear. The pulse is rapid and blood pressure is normal. The sputum is usually viscid and difficult to expectorate. If the attack has been present for many hours or days without remission despite treatment, the patient has status asthmaticus. This is often associated with signs of exhaustion and dehydration. Tachycardia is the rule and if greater than 130 per minute, indicates severe hypoxemia. Rarely, in patients with very prolonged airflow obstruction, edema of the feet and ankles may occur without other clinical evidence of heart failure.

## DIAGNOSIS

Essentials of diagnosis:
• Recurrent acute attacks of dyspnea, cough and mucoid sputum are usually accompanied by wheezing.
• Prolonged expiration with generalized wheezing and musical rales.
• Bronchial obstruction reversible by drugs.

## TREATMENT

**I. Treatment in Western medicine.**

Epinephrine and intravenous aminophylline are the drugs of choice for the emergency management of acute asthma. However, for status asthmaticus or for acute attacks in epinephrine-resistant patients, the adrenal corticosteroids are usually necessary. Intravenous hydrocortisone and methylprednisolone are the preparation of choice. But epiniphrine should not be used in patients with hypertension or angina or in elderly patients.

A. Epinephrine (1:1000), 0.2-0.5 ml subcutaneously, is the initial drug of choice and may be repeated every 1 to 2 hours.

B. Aminophylline, 250mg in 10-20ml saline administered slowly and intravenously, can be prescribed if epinephrine is not effective. Oral dose of aminophylline is usually 100mg, 4 times daily.

C. Isoproterenol (1:200), 1-2 inhalations from a hand nebulizer every 30 to 60 minutes, is most effective in mild attacks.

D. Corticosteroid drugs are most effective in severe attacks that do not respond satisfactorily to the bronchodilators.

E. Prednisone is given 40-60mg/d in divided doses and gradually reduced to nil over 7 to 10 days.

## II. Management in traditional Chinese medicine.

### 1. Herb therapy

A. Wind cold type. The patient complains of chills, headache, nasal obstruction, thin nasal discharge, rapid shallow breathing and flapping of alae nasi. His mouth is kept open with difficulty in breathing and the shoulders become elevated and he is unable to lie flat. On examination, the tongue is found covered with white coating and the pulse is smooth and rapid.

The principle of management is to remove the wind, expel the cold, eliminate the phlegm and calm asthma. The formula of first choice is Xiao Qin Lun Tang Jia Jian.

Constituents:

Chinese ephedra 6g
Cassia (twig) 10g
Wildginger (whole plant) 2g
Pinellia (tuber) 12g
Fruit of Chinese magnoliavine 12g
Dried ginger (rhizome) 10g
Blackberry lily (rhizome) 10g
Root of herbaceous peony 12g
Bulb of fritillary 10g
Tatarian aster (root) 24g
Common coltsfoot flower 10g
Apricot kernel 12g

Decoction and dosage. All the above herbs make a dose and six to ten doses are prescribed with one dose daily. Each dose is simmered twice and then the broth of each mixed, half of the mixed broth each time, twice a day.

B. Pulmonary heat type. This type is characterized by cough with yellowish mucoid phlegm and rapid shallow breathing which is performed with effort or even with flapping of alae nasi. The mouth of the patient is kept open and the shoulders become elevated and he may or may not have fever. On examination, the tongue is found with yellow coating and the pulse is rapid and smooth.

The principles for treatment are eliminating the phlegm, clearing heat, calming cough and relieving asthma. Ma Xing Shi Gan Tang Jia Jian is the best formula for the disorder.

Constituents:

Chinese ephedra 10g
Apricot kernel 12g
Gypsum 15-30g

Honeysuckle flower 15-30g
Weeping forsythia 15-30g
Blackberry lily (rhizome) 10g
Bulb of fritillary 10g
Root-bark of white mulberry 30g
Perillaseed 15g
Seed of welsh-onion 18g
Root of purple-flowered peucedanum 15g
Licorice root 6g

Decoction and dosage is the same.

C. Phlegm stagnation type. The typical features of this type are feelings of suppression in the chest and abundant thin whitish phlegm which is easily coughed up. On examination, the tongue is found covered with slippery and mucoid white coating and the pulse is slippery.

The basic principles for treatment are drying the damp, eliminating phlegm, relieving asthma and clearing cough. San Zhi Yang Qin Tang Jia Jian is the best formula.

Constituents:

Perillaseed 12-20g
White mustard seed 10g
Chinese radish seed 18g
Seed of welsh-onion 12-20g
Tatarian aster (root) 15-30g
Common coltsfoot flower 10g
Apricot kernel 12g
Bulb of fritillary 10g
Root of purple-flowered peucedanum 15g
Root-bark of white mulberry 15-30g
Root of the narrow-leaved polygala 12g
Dried old orange peel 12g
Pinellia (tuber) 12g

Decoction and dosage is the same.

Some ready made herb tablets such as Hai Zhu Chuan Xi Di Tablet are also effective for the illness. And Jin Kui Shen Qi Pills and Wu Zi Bu Shen Pills are also advisable for invigorating the vital portal at interim phase, according to the theory of traditional Chinese medicine that asthma is related to the deficiency of pulmonary and renal vital energy.

*2. Acupuncture therapy*

A. For wind cold type.
Points: B13 Feishu, L7 Lieque and LI4 Hegu.
B. For pulmonary heat type.
Points: S40 Fenglong, CV22 Tiantu, L5 Chize and Dingchuan Pt (extra).
C. For phlegm stagnation type.
Points: B13 Feishu, L9 Taiyuan, S36 Zusanli, B23 Shenshu, GV4 Mingmen and

CV Tanzhong.

Method: All the points are punctured with strong stimulation and the needles are retained for 20 to 30 minutes.

3. *Ear acupuncture therapy*

This therapy is given during the acute attacks.

Points: Lung Pt, Kidney Pt, Adrenal Gland Pt, Sympathetic Never Pt and Asthma Pt.

Method: Each time two or three of the above points are punctured and the needles are retained for 30 to 60 minutes. Each course includes ten to fifteen punctures and the treatment is ceased for 3 to 5 days between courses.

When combined together, the above therapies are very effective for asthma. When administered separately, Western medicine is good for relieving the attacks at acute stage and traditional Chinese medicine is more advisable for chronic cases. Acupuncture offers a quick relief to the attacks of asthma at acute stage.

# 4. PNEUMOCOCCAL PNEUMONIA

## GENERAL CONSIDERATION

Pneumococcal pneumonia, an inflammatory process in the lung parenchyma, is an acute bacterial infection of the lungs. It is caused by pneumococcus and characterized clinically by an abrupt onset with rigor, fever, chest pain, cough and blood sputum.

Pneumococcal pneumonia may occur at any season, but is most common during winter and early spring when viral respiratory infections are most prevalent.

The pneumococcus accounts for 60-80% of community-acquired bacterial pneumonia. These bacteria frequently are in the normal flora of the respiratory tract. The development of pneumonia therefore usually is attributed to the impairment of natural resistance. Conditions leading to aspiration of secretions include suppression of the cough or epiglottic reflex, impairment of upward migration of mucous sheets (propelled by cilia) and impairment of alveolar phagocyte function. Among conditions that predispose to pneumonia are viral respiratory diseases, malnutrition, exposure to cold, noxious gases, alcohol intoxication, depression of cerebral functions by drugs and cardiac failure. Pulmonary consolidation may be in one or more lobes or may be patchy in distribution.

In traditional Chinese medicine, this disorder is termed "Seasonal Disease," but the symptoms are equal to those of wind and warm symptom complex and winter fever or suppurative infections of the lungs and are thought to belong to acute febrile disease caused by pathogenic wind and warm factors in spring and winter or caused by different warm pathogenic factors in different seasons.

## CLINICAL MANIFESTATIONS

Victims of pneumococcal pneumonia are often found seriously ill. The onset is usually sudden with shaking chills, "stabbing" chest pain (exaggerated by respiration but sometimes referred to the shoulder, abdomen or flank), high fever, cough and "rusty" sputum and occasionally vomiting.

The patient appears severely ill with marked tachypnea (30-40%/min) but no orthopnea. Respirations are grunting and the patient often lies on the affected side in an attempt to splint the chest. Herpes simplex facial lesions are often present.

Initially, chest excursion is diminished on the involved side. Breath sounds are suppressed and fine inspiratory rales are heard. Later, the classic signs (absent breath sound, dullness, etc.) of consolidation appear. A pleural friction rub or abdominal distention may be present. During resolution of the pneumonia, the signs of consolidation are replaced by rales. Physical findings are often inconclusive and repeated x-ray examination is helpful. Constant features of the disease are fever and toxemia with the temperature usually ranging between 103 and 106 F. During the febrile period complaints of malaise, anorexia, weakness, myalgia and general prostration are extremely common.

## DIAGNOSIS

Essentials of diagnosis:

• Sudden onset of shaking chills, fever, chest pain and cough with rust-coloured sputum.

• X-rays show infiltration which is often lobar in distribution but sometimes can also be patchy.

• Pneumococci are present in the sputum and often in the blood.

• Leukocytosis.

• Newly-contracted acute febrile diseases or seasonal diseases including the wind and warm symptom complex and winter fever or suppurative infections of the lungs in traditional Chinese medicine.

## TREATMENT

### I. Treatment in Western medicine.

A blood culture and a good sputum specimen for smear and culture should always be obtained before treatment is started. The dosage and route of administration of antimicrobial drugs are influenced to some extent by the clinical severity of the disease, the presence of unfavourable prognostic signs and the presence of complications.

*1. Antibacterial therapy*

A. Penicillin G is the drug of choice. It is given initially in dosages ranging from 800,000 units of procaine penicillin every 12 hours intramuscularly for moderate illness to 1 million units of aqueous penicillin G every 4 hours rapidly into an intravenous infusion in severe cases.

B. Sulfonamides are not in favor now because the therapeutic response is slower than with penicillin. However, sulfisoxazole diolamine or sodium sulfadiazine 4 to 6 grams intravenously, followed by maintenance doses intravenously or orally is adequate (if not optimal) for many cases of pneumococcal pneumonia.

2. *General supportive treatment*

A. Ventilation and oxygenation. An adequate airway must be maintained, if necessary, by tracheal suction, endotracheal tube or trachostomy. Oxygen may be supplied by nasal catheter, soft rubber mask or oxygen tent.

B. Management of shock and pulmonary edema. Shock and pulmonary edema are the most frequent causes of death in pneumonia. Oxygen administration tends to prevent pulmonary edema and impending right heart failure must be managed and digitalization is urgent.

C. Management of toxic delirium. Toxic delirium occurs in any severe pneumonia and may be particularly difficult to manage in alcoholics. Delirium, anxiety and restlessness during waking hours may be treated with diazepam 5mg or chlordiazepoxide 10mg or phenobarbital 15 to 30 grams orally 4 to 6 times daily. Pentobarbital 0.1g or flurazepam (Dalmane) 30mg at bedtime helps to ensure adequate rest.

D. Fluids. Patients with pneumococcal pneumonia may perspire profusely and lose much fluid and salt. Sufficient fluid must be given to maintain a daily urinary output of at least 1500ml. Electrolytes must be kept in balance.

E. Pleuritic pain. For mild pain, spray ethyl chloride over the area of greatest pain for about 1 minute or inject a local anesthetic to anesthize the involved dermatomes to provide temporary relief.

Codeine phosphate 15-30mg may be given as necessary for pain. For very severe pain, use meperidine 50-100mg subcutaneously or morphine sulfate 10-15mg subcutaneously.

## II. Treatment in traditional Chinese medicine.

*Herb therapy*

Pneumococcal pneumonia which is termed Heat Disease in traditional Chinese medicine and is divided into three types.

A. The *wei* (defense) phase of the lung. The clinical features at early stages are chills and fever, thirst, perspiration, cough and headache with thin white or yellowish coating of the tongue and superficial and rapid pulse.

The general rule of treatment is to use drugs with cold property to treat external symptom complex.

The best formula is Yin Xiao San Jia Jian.

Constituents:

Honeysuckle flower 15-30g
Weeping forsythia 15-30g
Bamboo leaves 10g
Schizonepeta tenuifolia 12g
Achene of great burdock 10g
Peppermint 10g
Common reed rhizome 30g
Root of balloonflower 12g
Root of Zhejiang figwort 15-30g

Tuber or dwarf lilyturf 18g
Fresh or dried root of rehmannia 18g
Gypsum 30-60g
Licorice root 6g

Decoction and dosage. All the above herbs make a dose and six to ten doses are prescribed with one dose daily. Each dose is simmered twice and then the broth of each mixed, half of the mixed broth each time, twice a day.

B. Excessive heat type. The chief symptoms of the pathologic manifestations of extreme excesses of internal heat are high fever, anxiety, profuse sweating, thirst, flushed face, deep coloured urine, constipation, cough and yellowish and dry coating of the tongue, and full and large pulse.

The general rule of treatment with Chinese herbal decoction is to purify the Qi with pungent and cold drugs.

The formula of first choice is Ma Xing Shi Gan Tang Jia Jian.
Constituents:

Chinese ephedra 10g
Apricot kernel 12g
Gypsum 30-60g
Root-bark of white mulberry 30g
Root of purple-flowered peucedanm 15g
Tatarian aster 24g
Common coltsfoot flower 10g
Tendril-leaved fritillary bulb 10g
Cordate houttuynia 30-60g
Skullcap (root) 10g

Decoction and dosage is the same.

C. Suppurative infections of the lungs. Patients with this type of disorder have suppuration, cough and foul-smelling of the sputum. He may or may not have high fever. Yellow coating of the tongue and large full pulse are present.

The general rule for treatment with Chinese herbal decoction is to dissipate heat and to detoxify the lung.

The effective formula is Qie Jing Wei Jing Tang.
Constituents:

Common reed rhizom 30g
Cordate houttuynia 30-60g
Skullcap (root) 10g
Root-bark of white mulberry 30g
Apricot kernel 12g
Root of purple-flowered peucedanum 15g
Root of balloonflower 12-15g
Chinese goldthread (rhizome) 6-10g
Dandelio 30g
Herba patrinia 30g
Peach kernel 12g

Sargentgloryvine stem 30g
Mother chrysanthemum 15g

Decoction and dosage is the same.
Antibacterial therapy is more effective than herbal therapy, but when combined, the result would be far more satisfactory than that of either of the two.

# Chapter II
# DISEASES OF THE HEART AND THE BLOOD VESSELS

## 1. ANGINA PECTORIS

### GENERAL CONSIDERATION

Angina pectoris is usually due to an arteriosclerotic heart disease, but in rare instances it may occur in the absence of a significant disease of the coronary arteries as a result of coronary spasm, stenosis or insufficiency, syphilitic aortitis, increased metabolic demands as in hyperthyroidism or after thyroid therapy, marked anemia or paroxysmal tachycardias with rapid ventricular rates. The underlying mechanism is a discrepancy between the myocardial demands for oxygen and the amount delivered through the coronary arteries.

Symptmatically, the condition equals "Chest Bi" (stagnant cardiac blood) and Zi Xin Tong in traditional Chinese medicine and is usually thought to be caused by eating too much heavy and fattening food and delicious drinks.

### CLINICAL MANIFESTATIONS

The distribution of the distress may vary widely in different patients, but is always the same for each individual. In 80 to 90% of cases the discomfort is felt behind or slightly to the left of the sternum. When it begins farther to the left or uncommonly on the right, it characteristically moves centrally and is felt deep in the chest. Although angina may radiate to any segment from C8 to T4, it radiates most often to the left shoulder and upper arm, frequently moving down the inner volar aspect of the arm to the elbow, forearm, wrist, or the fourth and fifth fingers. Radiation to the right shoulder and distally is less common, but the characteristics are the same. Occasionally, angina may be referred to or felt initially in the lower jaw, the base or back of the neck, the interscapular area or high in the left back.

Patients often do not refer to angina as a "pain" but as a sensation of squeezing, burning, pressing, choking, aching, bursting, "gas", or tightness. The diagnosis of angina pectoris is strongly supported if 0.4mg of nitroglycerin invariably shortens an attack and if that amount taken immediately before exertion invariably permits greater exertion before the onset of angina or prevents angina entirely. Angina most commonly occurs during walking, especially up an incline or a flight of stairs.

Electrocardiography is normal in over one-fourth of patients with angina on that resting condition. It can be examined by exercise stress test, usually it shows patterns of left ventricular hypertrophy. Old myocardial infarction or non-specific ST-T changes also can be examined by radioisotope studies and some patients need examination by coronary angiography and left ventricular angiography.

## DIAGNOSIS

Essentials of diagnosis.

• Squeezing or pressurelike pain, retrosternal or slightly to the left, that appears quickly during exertion, may radiate in a set pattern and subside with rest.

• Seventy percent have diagnostic electrodiographic abnormalities after mild exercise; the remaining thirty percent have normal tracings or nondiagnostic abnormalities.

## TREATMENT

### I. Treatment in Western medicine.

A. Nitroglycerin is the drug of choice; it acts in about 1 to 2 minutes. As soon as the attack begins, place one fresh 0.3mg tablet under the tongue and allow it to dissolve.

B. Amyl nitrite, 1 pearl crushed and inhaled, acts in about 10 seconds.

C. Sublingual nifedipine, 10 to 20mg, may rapidly relieve angina, especially if spasm is the cause.

D. Oral isosorbide dinitrate, 2.5 to 10mg, 3 or more times daily.

E. Beta-blocking agents:

Propranolol (Inderal), 10 to 80mg, 3 to 4 times daily by mouth.

F. Platelet-inhibiting agents:

Aspirin, 0.3g/per day.

G. Inhibitors of the calcium slow-channel ionicflux:

Nifedipine, 10 to 20mg, 3 times daily by mouth is often helpful, especially when the patient suffers from hypertension.

H. General measures:

The patient must avoid all habits and activities known to bring on an attack. Most patients with angina do not require prolonged bed rest, but rest and relaxation are beneficial. Adequate mental rest is also important. Obese patients should be placed on a reducing diet and their weight brought to normal or slightly subnormal levels. Use of tobacco should be stopped or avoided because it produces tachycardia and elevation in blood pressure and because cigarette smoking has been shown to be a risk factor in coronary heart disease.

### II. Treatment in traditional Chinese medicine.

*1. Herb therapy*

A. For angina pectoris caused by stagnation of vital energy (qi) and blood. In this type the patients often feel squeezing, burning, pressing, choking, aching, bursting of the left of the sternum, radiating most often to the left shoulder and the upper arm, with distress of the chest, cold limbs, cyanosis, deep and rapid pulse and purple colour of the tongue.

The rule of treatment with herbs is to eliminate stagnation and activating blood with Tiao Heng Shi Wo Tang Jia Jian.

Constituents:

Milk veteh 35g
Chinese angelica  25g
Unpeeled root of herbaceous peony  25g
Chuanxiong 15g
Peach kernel  10g
Safflower 10g
Cattail pollen 12g
Faeces of flying squirrel 12g
Corydalis turtschaninovii 12g
Root of red rooted salvia  30g
Root of pseudo-ginseng 3g
Licorice root  6g
Cassia 12g

Decoction and dosage. Put all the above herbs together to be simmered twice and then the broth of each mixed, half of the mixed broth each time, twice a day.

B. For Chest Bi type. This symptom complex, due to the interference with the flow of the Yang Qi and the stagnation of the phlegm and the damp pathogen in the chest, chiefly manifests upper back pain, feeling of suffocation in the chest, shortness of breath, deep and rapid pulse, and purple colour of the tongue.

The rule of treatment with Chinese herbs is to clear the stagnation of the phlegm and invigorate the Yang with Gua Wei Jiu Bai Tang Jia Jian.

Constituents:

Mongolian snake gourd 25g
Onion bulb 15g
Milk veteh  35g
Chinese angelica  25g
Root of red rooted salivia  25g
Safflower 12g
Corydalis turtschaninovii 12g
Nutgrass flatsedge 15g
Root-tuber of aromatic turmeric  12g
Dried green orange peel 12g
Pinellia 12g
Fruit of immature citron or trifoliate orange  15g
Licorice root  6g

Decoction and dosage is the same.

*2. Acupuncture therapy*
Main points: B44 Shentang and P6 Neiguan.

Auxiliary points: B15 Xinshu, B14 Juejinshu, P5 Jianshi, H5 Tongli and H7 Shenmen.

Method: First puncture the left B44 Shentang superficially with strong stimulation. Then, 1 or 2 of each of the main and auxiliary points are punctured with either moderate or strong stimulation. The needles are retained for 20 to 30 minutes and the therapy is given once daily.

Note: Experiments show that acupuncture can reduce the left ventricular end-diastolic pressure through improving microcirculation, reducing coronary resistance, increasing coronary flow and the supply of oxygen to cardiac muscle, and reducing the myocardial consumption of oxygen.

*3. Point injection therapy*

Points: B15 Xinshu, B44 Shentang, CV17 Shanzhong, S16 Yingchuang, S18 Rugen, P3 Quze, S36 Zusanli and P5 Jianshi.

Drugs: 5% Chinese angelica solution, 10% salvia miltiorrhiza solution, 10% spatholobus suberectus solution and Vitamin C.

Method: Any of the above drugs can be prescribed and one point in the chest, back, upper limb and lower limb is injected with 0.5 to 1 millilitre of the selected solution. The therapy is given once daily and a course includes ten injections.

*4. Ear-acupuncture therapy*

Points: Heart Pt, Kidney Pt, Shenmen Pt, Subcortex Pt and Adrenal Pt.

Method: All the above points are punctured with strong stimulation and the needles are retained for 30 to 60 minutes. The therapy is given once daily and a course includes ten punctures.

# 2. PULSELESS DISEASE

## GENERAL CONSIDERATION

Pulseless disease, most frequent in young women, is an occlusive polyarteritis of unknown causes with a special predilection for the branches of the aorticarch. It occurs most commonly in orientals.

Pulseless disease is an autoimmune disease which concerned with immune complex deposits, usually caused by septicemia, by tuberculosis or syphilis, or may be involved in rheumatic fever and in rheumatoid disease.

Based on the symptoms, the disease is classified into blood vessel Bi category in traditional Chinese medicine.

## CLINICAL MANIFESTATIONS

Manifestations depend upon the vessels involved. In the early stages of the disease, dyspnea, cough and edema may be present and disappear later. Localized pain over the affected arteries, loss of arterial pulse, fever, dizziness, syncope, headache and impaired vision with claudication in the upper or lower extremities are common, particularly in slight anemia.

Most patients have an increased erythrocyte sedimentation rate and creactive protein is present. Aortographic studies are essential in confirming the diagnosis. In some cases, aortography may show localized aneurysms.

## TREATMENT

### I. Treatment in Western medicine.

A. Prednisone, 10mg 3 times daily, can provide remission in most patients, but may be of no effect at all in few cases. When the condition is improved, the doses must be gradually decreased.

B. Cyclophosphamidum, 1 to 4mg/kg/day, can be administered orally or intramuscularly. The side effects such as marrow depression, hemuresis, impairment of the liver, gastrointestinal reaction and impairment of the oophoron must be prevented and considered.

C. Combined administration of prednisone and cyclophosphamidium in small dose can decrease drug toxicity.

Other drugs such as indomethacinum, phenybutazonum, aspirinum are also advisable.

### II. Treatment in traditional Chinese medicine.

*1. Herb therapy*

A. For the type of Qi deficiency with blood stasis. In this type, the patient have claudication in the upper or lower extremities, dizziness, slight anemia, syncope, loss of arterial pulse and pale tongue. The general rule for treatment is to reinforce Qi and activate the blood. The commonly used formula is Bu Yang Huan Wu Tang Jia Jian.

The constituents are:

Milk veteh 60g
Dangshen  30g
Chinese angelia 15g
Herba siphonostegiae 30g
Chuanxiong  15g
Unpeeled root of herbaceous peony  15g
Cassia  15g
Peach kernel  10g
Safflower  10g
Earth-worm  10g
Root of pseudo-ginfeng  2g
Longspur epimedium 24g
Saline cistanche  15g
Mankshood (root) 9g

Decoction and dosage. All the above herbs make a dose and each dose is simmered twice and then the broth of each mixed, half of the mixed broth each time, twice a day.

B. For the type of fire-toxins and stagnant blood. The clinical features of this type are fever, localized pain over the affected arteries, loss of arterial pulse, headache, dizziness, syncope, impaired vision with claudication in the upper or lower extremities, rapid pulse, redness of the tongue with yellow coating. The treatment is centered on dissipating heat and detoxifying and activating blood with Si Miao Yun An Tang Jia Jian.

The constituents are:

Honeysuckle flower 30g
Weeping forsythia (fruit) 30g
Root of Zhejiang figwort  30g
Sargentgloryvine stem  30g
Fresh or dried rehmannia 30g
Giant knotweed  30g
Chinese angelica 20g
Unpeeled root of herbaceous peony 25g
Licorice root  6g
Safflower  12g
Peach kernel 12g

Decoction and dosage is the same.

*2. Acupuncture therapy*

Points: LI11 Quchi and LI4 Hegu for pain in the arm; S36 Zusanli and G39 Xuanzhong for pain in the leg; Taiyang (extra) for headache and B1 Jingming for impaired vision.

Method: The puncture is moderate and the needles are retained for 20 minutes. The therapy is given once daily.


# 3. THROMBOPHLEBITIS OF THE SUPERFICIAL VEINS

## GENERAL CONSIDERATION

Superficial thrombophlebitis may occur spontaneously, as in pregnant or post-partum women or in individuals with varicose veins or thromboangiitis obliterans; or it may be associated with trauma, as in the case of a blow to the leg or following intravenous therapy with irritating solutions. In the migratory or recurrent form, thromboangiitis should be suspected. It may also be a manifestation of abdominal malignancy such as carcinoma of the pancreas or may be its earliest sign. The long saphenous vein is most often involved. Superficial thrombophlebitis may be associated with occult deep vein thrombosis in about 20% of cases. Pulmonary emboli are infrequent but do occur.

Short-term plastic venous catheterization of superficial arm veins is now in routine use. The catheter should be observed daily for signs of local inflammation. It should be removed if a local reaction develops in the vein and in any case it should be removed in 48 hours. If further intravenous therapy is necessary, a new catheter may be inserted in a new vein. Serious septic complications can occur if these rules are not followed. The steel intravenous needles with the anchoring flange (butterfly needle) is less likely to be associated with phlebitis and infection than the plastic.

According to the symptoms, the condition is termed vascular Bi, caused by a relative excess of the pathogenic heat factors.

## CLINICAL MANIFESTATIONS

The patients usually experience a dull pain in the region of the involved vein. Local findings consist of induration, redness and tenderness along the course of a vein. The process may be localized, or it may involve most of the long saphenous vein and its tributaries. The inflammatory reaction generally subsides in 1 or 2 weeks; a firm cord may remain for a much longer period. Edema of the extremity and deep calf tenderness are absent unless deep thrombophlebitis has also developed. If chills and high fever develop, septic thrombophlebitis exists.

## DIAGNOSIS

Essentials of diagnosis:
- Induration, redness and tenderness along a superficial vein.
- No significant swelling of the extremity.

## TREATMENT

### I. Treatment in Western medicine.

If the process is well localized and not near the saphenofemoral junction. Local heat and bed rest with the leg elevated are usually effective in limiting thrombosis. Phenylbutazone(Butazolidin), 100mg orally 3 times daily for 5 days, may aid in the resolution of the inflammatory process but is contraindicated in individuals with peptic ulcer.

If the process is very extensive or is progressing upward toward the saphenofemoral junction, or if it is in the proximity of saphenofemoral junction initially, ligation and division of the saphenous vein at the saphenofemoral junction is indicated. The inflammatory process usually regresses following this procedure, though removal of the involved segment of vein (stripping) may result in a more rapid recovery.

Anticoagulation therapy is indicated if there is a rapid progress and extension into the deep system.

Septic thrombophlebitis requires excision of the involved vein up to its junction with an uninvolved vein in order to help the continued seeding of the blood with bacteria.

### II. Treatment in traditional Chinese medicine.

Vascular Bi is a blockage syndrome characterized mainly by the symptoms of the blood vessels. The chief manifestations are irregular fever, burning sensation of the skin, pain of the muscles of the joints and erythematous rash, redness and tenderness along the course of a vein, rapid pulse and yellow coating of the tongue.

A. Si Miao Yun An Tang Jia Jian.
Constituents:

Honeysuckle flower 40g
Weeping forsythia (fruit) 40g
Root of Zhejiang figwort 30g
Chinese angelica 30g
Skullcap 12g
Chinese goldthread 12g
Corktree 12g
Dandelion 30g
Chinese violet 30g
Unpeeled root of herbaceous peony 30g
Root-bark of peony 12g
Chuanxiong 20g
Root of red rooted salvia 30g
Fresh or dried rehmannia 30g
Buffalo horn 30g

Decoction and dosage. Put all the above herbs together to be simmered twice and then the broth of each mixed, half of the mixed broth each time, twice a day. Six doses are prescribed.

B. Rumex madaio Makino. Fresh leaves of rumex madaio makino are smashed for application on the affected region, 3 times daily, each 60 grams.

The above herb therapies are very effective for this condition.


# 4. THROMBOANGITIS OBLITERANS (TAD)
## (Buerger's Disease)

### GENERAL CONSIDERATION

Buerger's disease is an episodic and segmental inflammatory and thrombotic process of the arteries and veins, principally in the limbs. It is seen most commonly in men between ages 25 to 40 who smoke. The effects of the disease are almost solely due to ischemia, complicated in the later stages by infection and tissue necrosis. The inflammatory process is intermittent, with quiescent periods lasting weeks, months, or years.

The arteries most commonly affected are the plantar and digital vessels in the foot and those in the lower leg. The arteries in the hands and wrists may also become involved. Different arterial segment may become occluded in successive episodes; a certain amount of recanalization occurs during quiescent periods.

Superficial migratory thrombophlebitis is a common early indication of the disease.

The cause is not known, but alteration in the collagen in the vessels suggests that it may be a collagen disorder. Damage to the blood vessels by pathogenic cold and its invasion into the deep tissues cause swelling and pain of the foot.

In traditional Chinese medicine, the swelling and pain of the foot is thought to be the damage of the blood vessels by cold which passes through the skin and causes stasis of Qi in the vessels.

## CLINICAL MANIFESTATIONS

The signs and symptoms are primarily those of arterial insufficiency, and the differentiation from arteriosclerotic peripheral vascular disease may be difficult, however, the following findings suggest Buerger's disease.

A. The patient is a man between age 20 to 40 who smokes.

B. There is a history or finding of small, red, tender cords resulting from migratory superficial segmental thrombophlebitis, usually in the saphenous tributaries rather than the main vessel. A biopsy of such vein often gives microscopic proof of Bureger's disease.

C. Intermittent claudication is common and is frequently noted in the palm of the hand or arch of the foot. Rest pain is common and, when present, is persistent. It tends to be more pronounced than in the patient with atherosclerosis, numbness, diminished sensation and pricking and burning pains may be present as a result of ischemic neuropathy.

D. The digit or the entire distal portion of the foot may be pale and cold, or there may be rubor that may remain relatively unchanged by posture; the skin may not blanch on elevation and on dependency the intensity of the rubor is often more pronounced than that seen in the atherosclerotic group. The distal vascular changes are often asymmetric, so that not all of the toes are affected to the same degree. Absence or impairment of pulsations in the dorsalis pedis, posterior tibial, ulnar or radial artery is frequent.

E. Trophic changes may be present, often with painful indolent ulcerations along the nail margins.

F. There is usually evidence of disease in both legs and possibly also in the hands and lower arms. There may be a history or findings of Raynaud's phenomenon in the finger or distal foot.

G. The course is usually intermittent with acute and often dramatic episodes followed by rather definite remissions. When the collateral vessels as well as the main channels have become occluded, an exacerbation is more likely to lead to gangrene and amputation. The course in the patient with atherosclerosis tends to be less dramatic and more persistent.

## DIAGNOSIS

Essentials of diagnosis.

• Almost always in young men who smoke.

• Extremities involved with inflammatory occlusions of the more distal arteries, resulting in circulation insufficiency of the toes or fingers.

• Thrombosis of superficial veins may also accur.

• The course of the illness is intermittent and amputation may be necessary, especially if smoking is not stopped.

In traditional Chinese medicine, the condition is termed "Tuoju," which simply means that gangrene of the fingers or toes with excruciating pain at first, and after rather a long time necrosis and sloughing off of the skin, subcutaneous tissues, muscles and bones, resembling thromboangiitis obliteration.

## TREATMENT

### I. Treatment in Western medicine.

1. Smoking must be given up. The disease is almost sure to progress if this advice is not heeded.

2. Surgical measure.

A. Sympathectomy. Sympathectomy is useful in eliminating the vasospastic manifestations of the disease and aiding in the establishment of collateral circulation to the skin. It may also relieve the mild or moderate forms of rest pain. If amputation of a digit is necessary, sympathectomy may aid in healing of the surgical wound.

B. Arterial grafts. Arterial grafting procedures are seldom indicated in patients with Buerger's disease because they do not usually have significant occlusive disease in the iliofemoral region.

C. Amputation. The indications for amputation are similar in many respects to those outlined for the atherosclerotic group, although the approach should be more conservative from the point of view of preservation of tissue. Most patients with Buerger's disease who are managed carefully and stop smoking do not require amputation of the fingers or toes. It is almost never necessary to amputate the entire hand, but amputation below the knee is occasionally necessary because of gangrene or severe pain in the foot.

### II. Treatment in traditional Chinese medicine.

*1. Herb therapy*

A. For accumulation of cold and stasis of Qi.

The pain of the legs and toes of the patient is related to cold weather and intermittent claudication is common. The affected foot is pale and cold. Most patients are men and heavy smokers. The dorsal pulse of foot becomes weak or not felt. The rule of treatment is to eliminate the stagnant and activate the blood with Tao Huang Shi Wu Tang Jia Jian.

The formula is composed of:

Chinese angelica  25g
Unpeeled root of herbaceous peony 25g
Prepared rhizome of rehmannia rhizoma  12g
Chuanxiong  12g
Peach kernel  12g
Safflower  12g
Cassia  18g
Root of red rooted salvia  25g
Ox-knee 15g
Wildginger  2g
Milk veteh  30g

Dragon's blood  10g

Decoction and dosage. Each dose is simmered twice and the broth of each mixed, half of the mixed broth each time, twice a day.

B. For Damage to the muscles by heat.

The pain of the legs and toes of the patient is complicated with intermittent claudication and signs and symptoms such as redness, swelling and heat of the foot, gangrene of the fingers or toes with excruciating pain at first and necrosis and sloughing off of the skin, subcutaneous tissues, muscles and bones after a long time. The dorsal pulse of the foot is weak or may not be felt. The rule of treatment for this type is to dissipate heat and to detoxify the body with Si Miao Yun An Tang Jia Jian.

Constituents of the formula:

Honeysuckle flower 60g
Chinese angelica 30g
Root of Zhejiang fingwort 30g
Peach kernel 12g
Safflower  12g
Unpeeled root of herbaceous peony 30g
Chuanxiong 20g
Fresh or dried root of rehmannia 20g
Skullcap  10g
Corktree  10g
Chinese violet 30g
Weeping forsythia  30g
Patrinia villosa 30g

Decoction and dosage is the same.

*2. Acupuncture therapy*

Points: Sp4 Gongsun, G8 Shugu and Bafeng (extra).

Method: All the above points are punctured each time and the needles are retained for 20 minutes. The therapy is given once daily.

# Chapter III
# DISEASES OF
# THE ALIMENTARY TRACT

## 1. CHRONIC GASTRITIS

### GENERAL CONSIDERATION

Chronic gastritis is usually classified on the basis of mucosal histology and/or the anatomic portion of the stomach involved. Although endoscopic and radiologic criteria for classifying chronic gastritis have been reported, gastric mucosal biopsy is the most reliable means of diagnosis. Biopsies should be obtained from reliable means of diagnosis. Biopsies should be obtained from several different areas, since chronic gastritis may be a localized disease.

Histologically, chronic gastritis is divided into superficial gastritis, atrophic gastritis, and gastric atrophy. When inflammatory cells (neutrophils, lymphocytes, plasma cells, and a few eosinophils) are limited to the gastric pits and upper lamina propria, gastritis is classified as superficial. In atrophic gastritis, inflammatory cells invade deeper into the lamina propria and glandular epithelim. Lymphoid follicles may also be seen. As the disease progresses, thinning of the mucosa occurs with loss of glandular elements. In some patients intestinal metaplasia develops with loss of parietal and chief cells and development of goblet cells, absorptive cells, and intestinal villi. Finally, in patients with gastric atrophy, parietal and chief cells are absent, mucosal thickness is reduced markedly, and only a small number of inflammatory cells are present.

Chronic atrophy gastritis has been divided into Type A and Type B, based primarily on the anatomic portion of the stomach involved and the presence or absence of parietal cell antibodies. In Type A gastritis, the fundus and body of the stomach are involved, whereas the antrum is relatively normal. Parietal cell antibodies are found in a large percentage of patients, and pernicious anemia may develop. On the other hand, in Type B gastritis the antrum is involved primarily. Although inflammation is found frequently in the fundus and body, parietal cell antibodies do not occur.

In traditional Chinese medicine, there is no equivalent term for chronic gastritis and this condition is described as disharmony of the function and coordination of the liver and the stomach, due to stagnation of dampness caused by deficiency of the spleen.

## CLINICAL MANIFESTATIONS

The vast majority of persons with chronic gastritis do not have symptoms. Gastrointestinal symptoms, if they occur, may include anorexia, epigastric pressure and fullness, heartburn, nausea, vomiting, specific food intolerance, a peptic ulcer-like syndrome, and anemia or gross hemorrhage. Physical findings are often absent or consist only of mild epigastric tenderness.

## DIAGNOSIS

Essentials of diagnosis.
- Symptoms, if present, consist of vague, nondescript upper abdominal distress.
- Mild epigastric tenderness or no physical findings whatever.
- Gastric biopsy is the definitive diagnostic technique.

## TREATMENT

### I. Treatment in Western medicine.

The treatment of chronic gastritis, except in those cases associated with pernicious anemia or iron deficiency anemia, is not very successful. A peptic ulcer regimen-elimination of possible aggravating factors such as alcohol, salicylates and other nonsteroidal anti-inflammatory drugs and caffeine-anticholinergic drugs and mild tranquilizers may give symptomatic relief.

### II. Treatment in traditional Chinese medicine.

*1. Herb therapy*

A. For stagnation of dampness due to deficiency of the spleen and the pathologic changes due to the retention of water and transmissive functions of the spleen. The main symptoms are anorexia, epigastric distress, abdominal distension, loose stools, nausea, no thirst, or preference for hot drinks, general anasarca, lassitude and weakness, thick glossy coating of the tongue, slow and formicant pulse, etc. The most effective formula is Ping Wei San Jia Jian.

Constituents:

Chinese atractylodes 15g
Large-headed atractylodes 15g
Bark of official magnolia 12g
Dried old orange peel 12g
Pinellia 12g
Tuckahoe 15g
Wrinkled ianthyssop 15g
Fruit of hawthorn 30g
Medicated leaven 30g
Malt 30g
Fruit of citro or trifoliate 15g

Rhizoma xorydalis 10g
Dangshen 12g
Nutgrass 15g
Fructus amomi 12g

Decoction and dosage: All the above herbs make a dose and six to ten doses are prescribed with one dose daily. Each dose is simmered twice and then the broth of each mixed, half of the mixed broth each time, twice a day.

B. For depressed liver due to the deficiency of spleen. The typical symptoms of this type are hypochondriac pain, anorexia, mental depression, dizziness, weakness, loose stools, whitish tongue coating, stringy pulse, etc. The following formula is prescribed to reinforce and strengthen Qi and clean the liver.

Xiao Yao San Jia Jian.

Constituents:

Chinese angelica 15g
Unpeeled root of herbaceous peony 13g
Root of herbaceous peony  15g
Chinese thorowax 10g
Tuckahoe 10g
Large-headed atractylodes 15g
Nutgrass flatsedge 15g
Root-tuber of aromatic turmeris 12g
Rhizoma corydalis 10g
Zedoary turmeric 18g
Malt (baked)  30g
Licorice root 6g

Decoction and dosage is the same.

C. For retention of food in the stomach. Improper and irregular meals cause retention of foodstuff in the stomach and impair proper digestion, leading to such symptoms as distension and pain of the epigastrium, eructation, vomiting, anorexia, regurgitation of acid, thick and rough coating of the tongue. The pulse is usually smooth. The formula for this is Bao He Wan Jia Jian.

Constituents:

Fruit of hawthorn (baked) 30g
Medicated leaven (baked) 30g
Malt (baked) 30g
Weeping forsythia 20g
Chinese radish seed 15g
Dried old orange peel 12g
Membrane of chicken gizzard 10g
Pinellia 12g
Tuckahoe 10g
Betal nut 12g
Fruit of citron or trifoliate orange 15g
Licorice root 6g

Decoction and dosage is the same.

*2. Acupuncture therapy*

Main points: CV12 Zhongwan, P6 Neiguan, S36 Zusanli and B21 Weishu.

Auxiliary points: S25 Tianshu and CV6 Quchi for abdominal distention; B20 Pishu for indigestion.

Method: 3 or 4 of the main points are punctured with moderate stimulation. The auxiliary points are prescribed according to the symptoms. The needles are retained for 15 minutes and the therapy is given once daily.

*3. Ear-acupuncture therapy*

Points: Stomach Pt, Spleen Pt, Liver Pt, Sympathetic Nerve Pt and Shenmen Pt.

Method: All the above points are punctured once daily with moderate stimulation and the needles are retained for 30 to 60 minutes.

*4. Point injection therapy*

Points: B21 Weishu, B20 Pishu, B18 Ganshu, CV12 Zhongwan, S21 Liangmen, S36 Zusanli and Sp6 Sanyinjiao.

Drugs: Vitamin B.

Method: Each time 3 or 4 of the above points are injected with 0.5 to 1 millilitre of the above drug in each. The therapy is given once daily.


## 2. DUODENAL ULCER

### GENERAL CONSIDERATION

The incidence of duodenal ulcer has been declining at a rate of about 8% per year for the past decade, but it still remains a major health problem. Although the average age at onset is 33, duodenal ulcer may occur at any time from infancy to the later years. It is 4 times as common in males as in females. Occurrence during pregnancy is unusual.

Duodenal ulcer is 4 or 5 times as common as benign gastric ulcer. Morbidity due to peptic ulcer is a major public health problem.

About 95% of duodenal ulcers occur in the duodenal bulb or cap, i.e. the first 5cm of the duodenum. The remainders are between this area and the ampulla. Ulcers below the ampulla are rare. The ulceration varies from a few millimeter to 1-2cm in diameter and extends at least through the muscularis mucosae, often through to the serosa and into the pancreas. The margins are sharp, but the surrounding mucosa is often inflamed and edematous. The base consists of granulation tissue and fibrous tissue, representing healing and continuing digestion.

Gastralgia or pain of the epigastrium in traditional Chinese medicine equal to duodenal ulcer. It is thought to be caused by cold, retention, injuries and indulgency of foods or drinks.

### CLINICAL MANIFESTATIONS

Symptoms may be absent, or vague and atypical. In the typical case, pain is described as gnawing, burning, cramplike, or aching or as "heartburn"; it is usually mild or moderate, located over a small area near the midline in the epigastrium near the xiphoid. The pain may radiate below the costal margins into the back, or rarely to the right shoulder. Nausea may be present and vomiting of small quantities of highly acid gastric juice with little or no retained food may occur. The distress usually occurs 45 to 60 minutes after a meal; is usually absent before breakfast; worsens as the day progresses; and may be most severe between 12 midnight and 2 A.M. It is relieved by food, milk, alkalies and vomiting generally within 5 to 30 minutes.

Spontaneous remissions and exacerbations are common. Precipitating factors are often unknown but may include trauma, infections, or physical or emotional distress.

Signs include superficial and deep epigastric tenderness, voluntary muscle guarding, and unilateral (rectus) spasm over the duodenal bulb.

## DIAGNOSIS

Essentials of diagnosis in Western medicine.
- Epigastric distress 45 to 60 minutes after meals, or nocturnal pain, both relieved by food, antacids, or vomiting.
- Epigastric tenderness and guarding.
- Chronic and periodic symptoms.
- Gastric analysis shows acid in all cases and hypersecretion in some.
- Ulcer crater or deformity of duodenal bulb on X-ray or with oral endoscopy.

## TREATMENT

### I. Treatment in Western medicine.

A. General measures. The patient should be encouraged to have adequate rest and sleep, and it may sometimes be necessary to recommend 2 or 3 weeks' rest from work if that can be managed. The patient who must continue to work should be given careful instructions about the medical program. Arrangements should be made for rest and sufficient sleep. Anxiety should be relieved whenever possible.

Alcohol should be strictly forbidden. The patient should quit smoking if that can be done without too much distress.

The following drugs may aggravate peptic ulcer or may even cause perforation and hemorrhage: rauwolfia, salicytes, phenylbutazone, indomethacin and other non-steroidal antiinflammatory analgesics. They should be discontinued if possible.

B. Diet. All controlled clinical studies have documented that neither the type nor the consistency of diet will affect the healing of ulcers. The important principle of dietary management of peptic ulcer are as follows: (1) nutritious diet; (2) regular meals; (3) restriction of coffee, tea, cola beverages, decaffeinated beverages, and alcohol; and (4) avoidance of foods that are clearly known to produce unpleasant symptoms in a given individual.

In the acute phase, when there is partial gastric outlet obstruction, it is often useful to begin with a full liquid diet, provided that 1-hour postprandial gastric residuals are less than 100ml. Large amounts of milk and cream in the diet are associated with a striking increase in deaths from myocardial infarction in ulcer patients. Interval feedings should be avoided. Food of any type or consistency has been shown to markedly stimulate gastric acid in the stomach.

It is doubtful that any dietary measures other than elimination of known aggravating factors play a significant role in preventing ulcer recurrence.

C. Antacids. Antacids usually relieve ulcer pain promptly. Antacid dosage should be selected on the basis of neutralizing capacity. The response to antacids varies widely according to the preparation, the dosage, and the individual patient. Most tablet preparations are relatively ineffective and should not be given.

In order to be effective, antacids must be taken frequently. During the acute phase, a full dose 1 to 3 hours after meals and at bedtime should be sufficient. If pain relief is not achieved on this regimen, the stomach is emptying too rapidly or the patient is secreting more acid than the antacid can neutralize.

Magnesium hydroxide-aluminum hydroxide mixtures are effective and widely used antacids. The usual dosage is 15 to 30ml. When full therapeutic doses are given, the magnesium in the mixtures may produce diarrhea; it may be necessary to alternate with a straight aluminum hydroxide gel preparation, which tends to be constipating. Prolonged ingestion of aluminum hydroxide gels may lead to phosphate depletion and osteoporosis. Magnesium salts should be used cautiously in patients with renal insufficiency.

Calcium carbonate has an excellent neutralizing action and may be used at times when the magnesium-aluminum gel antacids are inadequate. Antacid mixtures containing aluminum hydroxide, calcium carbonate and magnesium hydroxide are avoidable, and the usual dosage is 15 to 30ml. A paradoxic calcium-induced gastric hypersecretion has been reported but probably has no clinical significance with this combination agent. However, when calcium carbonate alone is used, there may be hypercalcemia on its attendant complications.

D. Sucralfate (carafate). This nonabsorbable aluminum salt of sucrose octasulfate is a mucosal protective agent that has antipepsin activity and tends to adhere to areas of gastric duodenal mucosal injuries, e.g. ulcers. It is as effective with duodenal ulcer as antacids or $H_2$ receptor blockers and has the advantage of being nonsystemic. The only side-effect reported to date is mild constipation in about 5% of patients. Dosage is 1g 30 to 60 minutes before meals and at bedtime. Acid must be present for therapeutic effect, and, therefore, $H_2$ receptor blockers should not be used concomitantly. Antacids may be used when necessary but not within 1 hour of sucralfate.

E. Histamine $H_2$ receptors antagonist. The histamine $H_2$ receptor blocker cimetidine (Tagament) markedly inhibits gastric secretion stimulated by food, gastrin, histamine, and caffeine. The dosage is 300mg 4 times daily before meals and at bedtime. The dose must be reduced by one-half in patients with renal insufficiency.

The drug has been reported to be of value in benign gastric ulcer, peptic esophagitis, Zollinger-Ellison's syndrome and stress ulcerations. Studies comparing cimentidine and potent antacids have shown them to be equally effective. The drug is approved in the USA for short-term treatment of duodenal ulcer (6-8 weeks),

Zollinger-Ellison's syndrome and hypersecretory states such as systemic mastocytosis. Rare side-effects have included gynecomastia, galactorrhea, impotence, skin rashes, leukopenia, agranulocytosis, hepatitis, elevated serum creatinine, and decreased IgA and IgM. Of more concern are interactions between cimetidine and warfarin, theophylline, lidocaine, and other drugs, which occur via the p-450 cytochrome system of the liver.

Other $H_2$ receptor blockers are currently under investigation (e.g. ranitidine) and should be available soon.

F. Sedatives. Tense and apprehensive patients will usually benefit greatly from sedation. Hypnotic doses of the drugs may be necessary to ensure sleep.

G. Parasympatholytic (anticholinergic) drugs. Although the parasympatholytic drugs have been widely used over a long period of time for treatment of peptic ulcer, their effectiveness is questionable. Their usefulness is limited largely to the relief of refractory pain. The dosage necessary to produce significant gastric antisecretory effect may cause blurring of vision, constipation, urinary retention, and tachycardia. If patients have gastric retention, these drugs are contraindicated.

Note: Belladonna and other anticholinergic drugs should be avoided in patients with glaucoma, esophageal reflux, gastric ulcer, pyloric obstruction, cardiospasm, gastrointestinal hemorrhage, bladder neck obstruction, or serious myocardial disease.

a. Belladonna extract, 8 to 24mg, or atropine, 0.25 to 0.5mg, 20 to 30 minutes before meals and at bedtime with or without sedatives.

b. Synthetic parasympatholytics. Numerous proprietary tertiary and quaternary amines are available as belladonna or atropine substitutes. Although they do not have central nervous system side-effects, it is difficult to substantiate other therapeutic advantages. They are also more expensive.

## II. Treatment in traditional Chinese medicine.

### 1. Herb therapy

For stomach cold type. The chief symptoms of this type are watery vomitus, tastelessness, fondness of hot drinks, chilliness of epigastrium with fondness for hot fomentation and whitish moist coating of the tongue. The formula for this type is Li Zhong Tang Jia Jian.

Constituents:

Monkshood (root)  10g
Dried ginger 10g
Dangshen 15g
Large-headed atractylodes  15g
Ovodia fruit  10g
Fructus amomi 10g
Dried old orange peel 12g
Pinellia 12g
Tuckahoe  10g
Inkfish bone 18g
Chinese atractylodes  12g

Rhizoma corydalis 10g

Decoction and dosage: Put all the above herbs together to be simmered twice, then the broth of each mixed, half of the mixed broth each time, twice a day.

For gastric failure to transport downward. If the splenic Qi fails to function downward, various symptoms of retrogressive upward motion will occur. The abnormalities are usually belching, regurgitation of acid, nausea and gastric pain. The formula for this type is Xue Fu Hua Dai Chi Shi Tang Jia Jian.

Constituents:

Dangshen 15g
Large-headed atractylodes 15g
British inula flower 10g
Red ochre 10g
Chinese atractylodes 12g
Nutgrass flatsedge 15g
Semen coicis 10g
Dried old orange peel 12g
Pinellia  12g
Tuckahoe 10g
Licorice 6g

Decoction and dosage is the same.

For stasis of Qi and stagnant of blood type. This type is characterized by pain of the epigastrium, tenderness, occasional hematemesis and tarry stool, purple tongue and rapid pulse. The formula for this type is Shi Xiao San Jia Jian.

Constituents:

Cattail pollen 12g
Faeces of flying squirrel 12g
Rhizoma corydalis 10g
Root of pseudo-ginseng 2g
Zedoary turmeric  18g
Dried old orange peel 10g
Pinellia 10g
Skullcap  10g
Hyacinth bletilla  20g
Inkfish bone 20g
Licorice 6g

Decoction and dosage is the same.

*2. Acupuncture therapy.*

Points: B21 Weishu, B18 Ganshu, CV12 Zhongwan and S36 Zusanli.

Auxiliary points: S21 Liangmen, P6 Neiguan and Sp6 Sanyinjiao.

Method: 2 or 3 of each of the main and auxiliary points are punctured with either moderate or strong stimulation. The needles are retained for 20 minutes and the therapy is given once daily.

*3. Cupping therapy*

Cupping is applied with either large or medium-sized cups mainly on the upper abdomen, or the Back-shu points for 10 to 15 minutes.

*4. Ear acupuncture therapy*

Points: Stomach Pt, Sympathetic Nerve Pt, Subcortex Pt and Duodemun Pt.

Method: Select 2 or 3 of the above points for each treatment. The needles are retained for 15 to 30 minutes. A course includes ten treatments and between courses the treatment is ceased for 2 or 3 days.

# 3. DIARRHEA

## GENERAL CONSIDERATION

Diarrhea is defined as an increase in the frequency, fluidity and volume of bowel movements. Normal bowel function varies from individual to individual, and the definition of diarrhea must take this variation into account. Factors influencing stool consistency are poorly understood; water content is not the sole determinant, thus, the definition of diarrhea in a clinical sense is an increase in frequency or increased fluidity of bowel movements in a given individual. In pathophysiologic terms, diarrhea results from the passage of stools containing excess water, i.e. from malabsorption or secretion of water.

Most diarrheal states are self-limited and pose no special diagnostic problem. They are often due to dietary indiscretions or mild gastrointestinal infections. The following list of the causes of diarrhea is indicative of the extensive diagnostic evaluation that may be required in patients with unexplained, profound or chronic diarrhea.

The many causes for diarrhea may be briefly outlined as follows:

A. Functional disorders including adaptive colitis, allergy to ingested food and drugs, defective gastric or pancreatic digestion, defective absorption, vitamin deficiencies and abuse of cathartics.

B. Generalized disorder or disease affecting the intestine, including uremia, Graves' disease, Addison's disease, cardiac decompensation, portal hypertension, neurologic disease and poisoning with heavy metals.

C. Intrinsic disease of the intestine, due to: A. Specific viral, bacterial and fungal infection, protozoan, or metazoan parasites; B. Alterations in intestinal flora, antimicrobial therapy, fistula, blind loops, or small intestinal stasis; C: Nonspecific inflammatory disease such as regional enteritis or ulcerative colitis; or D. Benign or malignant tumors and other causes of partial intestinal obstruction.

In traditional Chinese medicine, diarrhea is thought to be caused by inability of the body to regulate water, resulting in stasis of dampness in the stomach and intestine, or in the spleen. In diarrhea, kidney, large intestine and liver are often involved.

## CLINICAL MANIFESTATIONS

With excess fecal water:

Osmotic diarrhea—Excess water—soluble molecules in the bowel lumen cause osmotic retention of intraluminal water.

Secretory diarrhea—Excessive active ion secretion by the mucosal cells of the intestine.

Deletion or interference with normal ion absorption—This is usually a congenital problem.

Exudative disease—Abnormal mucosal permeability with intestinal loss of serum proteins, blood, mucus or pus.

Impaired contact between intestinal chyme and absorbing surface—Rapid transit, short bowel syndromes.

Without excess fecal water—frequent, small, painful evacuations are usually a result of disease of the left colon or rectum.

In traditional Chinese medicine, diarrhea is divided into 5 types:

A. Heat diarrhea. Due to the invasion of a pathogenic heat factor into the large intestine. The chief symptoms are diarrhea with very foul mucoid stools, borborygmus, abdominal pains, burning sensation of the anus, scanty dark urine, thirst.

B. Cold diarrhea. Caused by an invasion of the pathogenic cold factor into the gastrointestinal tract. The chief symptoms are watery stools with indigested food, vague abdominal pain, pale urine.

C. Damp diarrhea. Characterized by a sense of heaviness of the body, chest distress, no thirst, little abdominal pain, loose stools, scanty dark urine, mucoid glossy coating of the tongue, etc.

D. Food diarrhea. Caused by improper or contaminated diet. Clinically it is manifested as belching, regurgitation of acid, poor appetite, distress of the chest and epigastrium, and abdominal pain followed and relieved by diarrhea.

E. Early morning diarrhea. This type of diarrhea occurs just before dawn and is caused by deficiency of the kidney-Yang.

## DIAGNOSIS

Specific diagnosis is based on careful examination of the diarrhea material for polymorphonuclear cells and bacteria and, if indicated, for parasites. This is best accomplished at sigmoidoscopy prior to preparation with a cleansing enema. Cotton swabs should not be used in making slides, as both polymorphonuclear cells and parasites cling to cotton. The presence of polymorphonuclear cells indicates an inflammatory process. Rectal biopsy prove helpful, particularly when entamoeba histolytica is being considered and there is colitis. These studies should be performed prior to barium studies and treatment.

## TREATMENT

### I. Treatment in Western medicine.

Culture for bacterial pathogens and examination of several stools for polymorphonuclear cells and parasites must be done before barium studies or treatment are begun.

*1. Correct physiologic changes induced by diarrhea*

Acid-base disturbance, fluid loss.

Electrolyte depletion.

Malnutrition, vitamin deficiencies.

Psychogenic disturbances.

*2. Diet*

For acute severe diarrhea. Food should be withheld for the first 24 hours or restricted to clear liquids—a physiologic glucose and salt solution, sipped slowly as needed to replace large fluid and electrolyte losses, may be especially useful in patients with severe watery diarrhea. Frequent small soft feedings are added as tolerated.

For chronic diarrhea. Chronic diarrhea is due to many causes. Nutritional disturbances range from none to marked depletion of electrolytes, water, protein, fat and vitamins. Treat specific disease when known. Give fat soluble vitamins when steatorrhea is present. Some patients are so ill that they require parenteral hyperalimentation, sometimes at home.

*3. Antidiarrhea agents*

A. Pepto-bismol. Give 30ml 3 to 6 times per day for symptomatic treatment of diarrhea.

B. Narcotic analogs. Avoid with possible acute infectious diarrhea, as they may worsen the course.

a. Lomotil (diphenoxylate with atropine). 2.5mg, 3 or 4 times daily as needed. It must be used cautiously in patients with advanced liver disease and in those who are addiction-prone or who are taking barbiturates.

b. Loperamide (imodium). 2mg 2 to 4 times daily is effective in acute and chronic diarrhea.

C. Narcotics. Narcotics must be avoided in chronic diarrhea and are preferably avoided in acute diarrheas unless there is intractable diarrhea. Vomiting and colic always exclude the possibility of acute surgical abdominal disease before administering opiates. Any of the following drugs can be given:

a. Paregoric, 4 to 8ml after liquid movements as needed or with bismuth.

b. Codeine phosphate. 15 to 65mg subcutaneously, if the patient is vomiting, after liquid bowel movements as needed.

c. Strong opiates. Morphine and hydromorphone should be reserved for selected patients with severe acute diarrhea who fail to respond to more conservative measures.

D. Anticholinergic drugs, particularly when used in combination with sedatives, exert a mild antiperistaltic action in acute and chronic diarrheas associated with anxiety and tension states. It may be necessary to administer the various drugs to a point near toxicity in order to achieve the desired effect.

Antidiarrheal drugs must be used with great caution in inflammatory bowel disease and amebiasis because of the risk of "toxic" dilatation of the colon. Unless diarrhea is severe, they should be avoided in bacillary dysentery, since they prolong the carrier state.

### 4. Psychotherapy

Many cases of chronic diarrhea are of psychogenic origin. A survey of anxiety-producing mechanism should be made in all patients with this complaint. Antidepressant drug therapy may be useful, particularly since many of these agents have an anticholinergic effect.

## II. Treatment in Chinese medicine.

### 1. Herb therapy

In traditional Chinese medicine, the condition is divided into five types, each of which is treated with different herbs.

A. For Chang Pi type. Chang Pi is an acute intestinal infection commonly seen in summer and autumn, and characterized by watery diarrhea, cramp of the gastrocnemius muscles of the leg due to excessive loss of water from severe vomiting and diarrhea, thirst, dark urine and profuse sweating, mucoid glossy coating of the tongue. The formula for this type is Qin Sao Wei Lin Tang Jia Jian.

Constituents:

Skullcap 10g
Root of herbaceous peony  30g
Chinese atractylodes 15g
Bark of official magnolia  10g
Dried old orange peel  12g
Pinellia 10g
Tuckahoe  30g
Umbellate pore 12g
Oriental water plantain 12g
Asiatic plantain 30g
Wrinkled leaven 12g
Leaf of purple perilla 12g

Decoction and dosage: All the above herbs make a dose and six to ten doses are prescribed with one dose daily. Each dose is simmered twice and then the broth of each mixed, half of the mixed broth each time, twice a day.

B. For Heat type. Heat type diarrhea is due to the invasion of a pathogenic heat factor into the large intestine. The chief symptoms are diarrhea with very foul mucoid stools, borborygmus, abdominal pains, burning sensation of the anus, scanty dark urine, thirst, tenesmus, yellow coating of the tongue, rapid pulse. The treatment is to dissipate heat with Ge Gen Qin Lian Tang Jia Jian.

Constituents:

Root of kudzuvine  15g
Skullcap 10g
Chinese goldthread 10g
Chinese pulsatilla 20g
Corktree 12g
Ash bark  12g
Purslane 30g

Fruit of hawthorn 30g
Betal nut 15g

Decoction and dosage is the same.

C. For food type. Food type diarrhea is caused by improper or contaminated diets, clinically it is manifested as belching, regurgitation of acid, poor appetite, distress of the chest and epigastrium, abdominal pain followed and relieved by diarrhea, thick coating of the tongue, etc. The treatment is intended to relieve food accumulation with Bao He Wan Jia Jian.

Constituents:

Fruit of hawthorn 30g
Medicated leaven 30g
Malt 30g
Weeping forsythia 15g
Chinese radish seed 18g
Dried old orange peel 12g
Pinellia  12g
Wrinkled leaven 12g
Membrane of chicken gizzard 10g
Rhubarb 6g

Decoction and dosage is the same.

D. For the type of deficiency of the spleen-Yang. The pathologic manifestations of the decline of splenic functions together with the cold syndrome. The main symptoms are distension, chilliness and pain of epigastrium, anorexia, loose stools or chronic diarrhea or chronic dysentery, cold limbs, pale tongue with whitish coating, empty and slow pulse, etc. The treatment is to warm and strengthen the spleen with Shen Lin Bai Su San Jia Jian.

Constituents:

Dangshen  12g
Large-headed atractylodes (baked) 30g
Chinese atractylodes 15g
Chinese yam rhizome 30g
Bean of white hyacinth dolichos  30g
Semen coicis 10g
Coix seed  30g
Hibdu lotus 12g
Dried old orange peel 12g
Pinellia 12g
Tuckahoe 30g
Fruit of hawthorn 30g
Medicated leaven 30g
Malt 30g
Monkshood (root) 10g
Wrinkled leaven 12g

Decoction and dosage is the same.

E. For the type of deficiency of kidney-Yang. The patients with this type of diarrhea always complain of diarrhea before dawn with chilliness of the abdomen, cold limbs, impaired appetite, chill and pain of the waist and knees, abdominal pain which can be relieved by discharge of the feces, pale tongue, small formicant pulse, etc. The treatment is to invigorate the kidney-Yang with Shi Sheng Wan Jia Jian.

Constituents:

Nutmeg 12g
Malaytea scurfpea 12g
Fruit of Chinese magnoliavine 12g
Evodia fruit 10g
Chinese Yam rhizome 30g
Chinese atractylodes 15g
Large-headed atractylodes 30g
Coix seed 30g
Bean of white hyacinth dolichos 30g
Bark of Chinese cassia tree 2g
Dried ginger 10g
Licorice root 6g

Decoction and dosage is the same.

In addition many ready made herb pills are also very effective for diarrhea.

*2. Acupuncture therapy*

Main points: S25 Tianshu, B25 Dachangshu and S36 Zusanli.

Auxiliary points: CV12 Zhongwan for cold-damp syndrome; S44 Neiting, Sp9 Yinlingquan and LI4 Hegu for damp-heat syndrome; B20 Pishu, Liv13 Zhangmen, Sp3 Taibai and CV12 Zhongwan for deficiency of the Yang and spleen.

Method: All the main points are punctured together with the auxiliary ones which are selected according to the symptoms. The puncture is moderate and the needles are retained for 20 minutes. The therapy is given once daily. Moxibustion is applied to GV20 Baihui to raise Qi of the spleen and stomach.

*3. Cutting therapy*

Points for cutting: B20 Pishu and B23 Shenshu.

Method: Carefully sterilize the skin of the points before infiltration anesthesia with 1 novocain. A longitudinal incision is conducted on the point and a little subcutaneous fatty tissue is removed. Then the cut is sutured and dressed. The stitch is removed a week later and the second therapy is given 2 or 3 weeks afterwards.

# 4. NONSPECIFIC ULCERATIVE COLITIS

## GENERAL CONSIDERATION

Ulcerative colitis is an inflammatory disease of the colon of unknown causes characterized by bloody diarrhea, a tendency to remissions and exacerbations and involvement mainly of the left colon. It is primarily a disease of adolescents and young adults but may have its onset in any age group.

The pathologic process is that of acute nonspecific inflammation in the colon, particularly the rectosigmoid area, with multiple irregular superficial ulcerations. Repeated episodes lead to thickening of the wall with scar tissue, and the proliferative changes in the epithelium may lead to polypoid structures. Pseudopolyps are usually indicative of severe ulceration. The cause is not known; it may be multiple.

The disease is usually called "dysentery," "damp-heat dysentery" or "bloody stool" in traditional Chinese medicine, and is thought to be caused by internal stasis of dampness and heat. The pathologic changes in which damp and heat pathogens stay deeply in the body. Thereby various manifestations of gastrosplenic dysfunctions may occur.

## CLINICAL MANIFESTATIONS

This disease may vary from mild cases with relatively minimal symptoms to acute and fulminating ones with severe diarrhea and prostration. Diarrhea is characteristic; there may be up to 30 or 40 discharges daily, with blood and mucus in the stool, or blood and mucus may occur without feces. Blood in the stool is the cardinal manifestation of ulcerative colitis. Constipation may occur instead of diarrhea.

Nocturnal diarrhea is usually present when daytime diarrhea is severe. Rectal tenesmus may be severe, and anal incontinence may be present. Cramping lower abdominal pain often occurs but is generally mild. Anorexia, malaise, weakness and fatigability may also be present. A history of intolerance to dairy products can often be obtained, and there is a tendency toward remissions and exacerbations.

Fever, weight loss and evidence of toxemia vary with the severity of the disease. Abdominal tenderness is generally mild and occurs without signs of peritoneal irritation. Abdominal distention may present in the fulminating form and is a poor prognostic sign. Rectal examination may show perianal irritation, fissures, hemorrhoids, fistulas and abscesses.

## DIAGNOSIS

Essentials of diagnosis in Western medicine.
• Bloody diarrhea with lower abdominal cramps.
• Mild abdominal tenderness, weight loss, fever.
• Anemia: No stool pathogens.
• Specific X-ray and sigmoidoscopic abnormalities.

X-ray findings: As shown by X-ray, the involvement may be regional or generalized and may vary from irritability and fuzzy margins to pseudopolyps, decreased size of colon, shortening and narrowing of the lumen, and loss of haustral markings. When the disease is limited to the rectosigmoid area, the barium enema may even be normal.

Sigmoidoscopic changes are present in over 95% of cases and vary from mucosal hyperemia, petechiae and minimal granularity in mild cases to ulceration and polypoid changes in severe cases. The mucosa, even when it appears grossly normal, is almost invariably friable when wiped with a cotton sponge. Colonoscopic examination may prove useful in defining the extent of ulcerative colitis and in permitting biopsy of radiographically suspect regions.

## TREATMENT

### I. Treatment in Western medicine.

Ulcerative colitis is a chronic disease characterized by recurrent exacerbations, varying degrees of damage to the colonic mucosa and complications both intestinal and extraintestinal. The treatment programs should attempt to: (1) terminate the acute attack; (2) prevent recurrent attacks; and (3) promote healing of the damaged mucosa. Long-term therapy may be modified by considerations relating to complications, e.g. carcinoma and ocular disease. Symptomatic remission should not be the only index of therapeutic response.

The choice and intensity of therapy should be determined by the clinical severity of the disease.

*1. Severe (Fulminant) disease*

A. Hospitalization. Hospitalization is indicated. Patients with severe disease may deteriorate rapidly with hemorrhage, perforation, toxic megacolon and sepsis developing over a short period of time.

B. General measures.

a. Restore circulating blood volume with fluids, plasma and blood as indicated.

b. Discontinue opiates and anticholinergics.

c. Correct electrolyte abnormalities.

d. Discontinue all oral intake. Institute nasogastric suction if the colon has become dilated.

C. Antimicrobial therapy. The clinical course of fulminant ulcerative colitis is associated with extensive necrosis of colonic mucosa and perforation with sepsis is not uncommon in this form of the disease. Intravenous antibiotics are given to these patients for presumed or potential sepsis. Ampicillin, cephalothin, cephapirin, chlorampnenical and gentamicine have been used singly or in combination.

D. Adrenocorticosteroids. Give intravenous hydrocortisone, 300mg daily, or prednisone, 60mg daily in divided doses at 6 to 8 hour intervals.

E. Surgery. If the patient with toxic colonic dilation does not improve within 8 to 12 hours, colonic resection is usually indicated. In those patients who have fulminant disease but are not toxic, intravenous therapy is continued for 5 to 7 days. If improvement occurs, oral therapy can be substituted. If the patient fails to respond or deteriorates, colectomy should be considered. Malnourished patients may be benefited by total parenteral nutrition during this phase.

*2. Moderate disease*

This group of patients has substantial evidence of activity, i.e. diarrhea, abdominal cramping, weight loss and anemia, and hospitalization should be advised, even though they are not toxic, i.e. they do not have severe hypoproteinemia, fever or leukocytosis.

A. Diet. Give no milk or milk products. All foods must be cooked.

B. Adrenocorticosteroids. Give prednisone, 20 to 60mg orally daily, and reduce by 5mg per week when there is clinical and sigmoidoscopic evidence of improvement. Hydrocortisone enemas, 100mg each night, may provide additional antiinflammatory effect.

C. Antimicrobial therapy. Sulfasalazine, 2 to 4g daily in divided doses, has been shown to be beneficial in reducing inflammation and in decreasing the frequency of recurrent attack in this form of the disease. It has been suggested that 5-aminosalicylic acid is the active moiety of sulfasalazine. Sulfasalazine has been shown to decrease the number and motility of sperms and increase the frequency of abnormal sperms. Infertility may occur during the treatment period.

3. *Mild disease*

These patients have minimal evidence of inflammatory bowel disease, i.e. asymptomatic rectal bleeding, minimal involvement by sigmoidoscopic examination, and on systemic signs of the disease.

A. Diet. Give no milk products.

B. Antimicrobial therapy. Sulfasalazine, 2 to 4g daily in divided doses as prolonged maintenance therapy.

C. Adrenocorticosteroids. Hydrocortisone enemas or suppositories, 100mg each night until lesion heals or disease has been stable for several months.

4. *Surgical measures*

Surgical excision of the colon is required for patients with refractory disease, severe extracolonic complications(growth suppression), prolonged widespread colon disease, massive hemorrhage, or extensive perirectal disease. The usual procedure is total colectomy with a permanent ileostomy. In some instances, the rectum may be preserved and a primary reanastomosis or subsequent reanastomosis carried out if the rectum appears normal or minimally involved.

All of these method may be effective to control symptoms in short-term, but recurrent rate is high. The course of treatment with these medicines is longer, and the side effect is marked. Some reports demonstrated that the effect was not satisfactory.

## II. Treatment in traditional Chinese medicine.

A. Enema with herb decoction. 75 to 100ml concentrated decoction of medicinal herbs is given to the patient once daily. A course includes 30 times and between courses there is an interval of 7 days.

For patients with nonspecific ulcerative colitis who have bloody pus, the following formula is prescribed.

Constituents:

Polygonum multiflorum  15g
Polygonum amplexicaule  15g
Limonium bicolour  30g
Field thistle  30g
Root of garden burnet (baked)  30g
Hyacinth bletilla (tuber) 15g

Rodgersia aesculifolia batal  15g
Copperleaf  30g

Decoction and dosage: All the above herbs make a dose and six to ten doses are prescribed with one dose daily. For patients with mucus stool, the following formula is prescribed.

Constituents:

Polugonum multiflorum  15g
Polygonum amplexicaule  15g
Hyacinth bletilla 12g
Climbing groundsel  30g
Licorice root 15g
Cortree (bark)  12g
Oldenlandia diffusa (wild.) Roxb  30g
Herba patriniae 30g

Decoction and dosage is the same.
B. Enema with a mixture of the following drugs:

Baiyao 0.4g
Berberine 1g
0.25% procain  20ml
0.9% Nacl sol  60ml

Dosage. Once daily and a course includes ten times.
C. Point injection therapy.
Points: S25 Tianshu, B20 Pishu, B21 Weishu and S36 Zusanli.
Drugs: Vit C 500mg.
Method: Each of the above points is injected with 0.5mg of Vitamin C and the therapy is given once daily.


# 5. VIRAL HEPATITIS

## GENERAL CONSIDERATION

Hepatitis A is a viral infection of the liver that may occur sporadically or in epidemics. The liver involvement is part of a generalized infection but dominates the clinical picture. Although transmission of the virus may occur by contaminated needles, it is usually by the fecal-oral route. The excretion of hepatitis A virus (HAV) as determined by immune electron microscopy of stool occurs up to 2 weeks prior to illness. HAV is rarely demonstrated in feces after the third week of illness. There is no known carrier state with HAV. Blood and stools are infectious during the incubation period (2 to 6 weeks) and early illness until peak transaminase levels are achieved. Although theoretically possible, the short duration of viremia makes posttransfusion hepatitis unlikely. In fact, posttransfusion hepatitis due to HAV has not been documented. Although the mortality rate with hepititis A is low, it may cause fulminant disease. The mortality rate (as with hepatitis B) appears to be age-related. Marmoset monkeys and chimpanzees appear to be the only susceptible animals; livers of infected marmoset monkeys have revealed the 27-nm particles.

An unequivocal diagnosis of HAV is established by demonstrating the hepatitis A virus antigen (HAAg) in the stool or the IgM antibody to hepatitis A in serum. The absence of HAAg in the stool does not rule out HAV infection.

Antibodies to type A hepatitis appear early in the course of the illness and tend to persist in the serum. Immune electron microscopy and radioimmunoassay detect both IgM and IgG antibodies and are positive soon after the onset of the illness. Immune adherence hemagglutination reflects an IgG response and is positive later in the course of the disease. Peak titers of IgG antibodies occur after 1 month of disease and may persist for years. Peak titers of IgG antibodies occur during the first week of clinical disease and disappear within an 8-week period; therefore measurement of these antibodies is an excellent test for demonstrating acute hepatitis A infection. The presence of anti-HAV activity indicates: (1) previous exposure to HAV; (2) noninfectivity; and (3) immunity to recurring HAV infection. It does not imply previous clinically apparent hepatitis, nor does it establish a relationship to ongoing liver disease unless seroconversion has been demonstrated.

The viral agent of hepatitis A is a small 27-nm RNA virus that belongs to the picornavirus group, which also includes poliomyelitis virus and coxsackie-virus. The agent is inactivated by ultraviolet light, by heating to 100 degrees centigrade for 5 minutes, and by exposure to 1:4000 formalin solution.

Hepatitis B is a viral infection of the liver usually transmitted by inoculation of infected blood or blood products. However, the antigen has been found in most body secretions, and it is known that the disease can be spread by oral or sexual contact. Hepatitis B virus (HBA) is highly prevalent in homosexuals and intravenous drugs abusers. Other group at high risk include patients and staff at hemodialysis centers, physicians, dentists, nurses and personnel working in clinical and pathologic laboratories. Approximately 5-10% of infected individuals become carriers, providing a substantial reservoir of infection. 40-70% of infants born to HBsAg-positive mothers will develop antigens to hepatitis B in the bloodstream. Fecal-oral transmission of virus B has also been documented. The incubation period of hepatitis B is 6 weeks to 6 months. Clinical features of hepatitis A and B are similar; however, the onset in hepatitis B tends to be more insidious.

Hepatitis B virus is pleomorphic and occurs in spherical and tubular forms of different sizes. The largest of these, the Dane particle, is thought to be the complete infectious virus. The 42-nm Dane particle is composed of a core (27-nm particle) found in the nucleus of infected liver cells, and a double-shelled surface particle found in the cytoplasm. The other particles form an excess coating of the virus and contain no nucleic acid.

There are 3 distinct antigen-antibody systems that relate to HBV infection. In addition, DNA polymerase activity can be measured as a sensitive index of viral replication and infectivity.

The surface antigen (HBsAg) is the antigen routinely measured in blood. HBsAg is unaffected by repeated freezing and thawing or by heating at 56 degrees centigrade overnight or at 60 degrees centigrade for 1 hour. It is inactivated by heating between 85 and 100 degrees centigrade for 15 to 30 minutes. HBsAg can exist in serum as 3 antigenically identical forms: (1) the outer coat of the intact Dane particle; (2) a spherical 22-nm particle; and (3) elongated tubular particles. The spherical and tubular particles do not contain nucleic acid and are not infectious. Four major antigenic subtypes of HBAg have been recognized. Subtyping of HBsAg if primarily of epidemiologic importance. The presence of GBsAg is the first manifestation of HBV infection occurring before biochemical evidence of liver disease. HBsAg persists throughout the clinical illness, persistence of HBsAg is usually associated with clinical and laboratory evidence of chronic hepatitis. The presence of HBsAg establishes infection with HBV and implies infectivity. Specific antibody to HBsAg (anti-HBs) occurs in most individuals after clearance of HBsAg. Anti-HBs is usually delayed after clearance of HBsAg. During this serologic gap, infectivity has been demonstrated. Development of anti-HBs signals recovery from HBV, noninfectivity, and protection from HBV infection.

Disruption of the Dane particle releases an antigenically distinct inner core structure (HBcAg). Antibodies against core antigen (anti-HBC) localize the core antigen primarily to the nucleus of infected human and primate liver cells. The core particles are not found in the serum. Core particles may be present in liver tissue in the absence of HBsAg, and recovery from HBV is complete only when the core particles are no longer detected in the liver. Anti-HBC appears shortly after HBsAg is detected and persists throughout the period of HBs antigenemia. It fills the serologic gap in patients who have cleared the HBsAg but have not demonstrated detectable amounts of anti-HBs. Anti-HBC can be found alone or in any combination with HBsAg or anti-HBs. Anti-HBC has been shown in all instances of acute HBV infection and appears simultaneously with the onset of clinical illness. Infectivity has been demonstrated in instances where donors are HBsAg-negative and positive for anti-HBC.

HBeAg is distinct from HBsAg. It is a soluble protein found only in HBsAg-positive sera. All patients with HBV infection demonstrate HBe antigenemia. HBeAg appears during the incubation period shortly after the detection of HBsAg and only during HBsAg reactivity. HBeAg may be a sensitive index of viral replication and infectivity. Anti-HBe is detected as early as the fourth week of illness. The clinical usefulness of this antigen-antibody system lies in its predictive value of infectivity.

DNA polymerase activity is first detectable at the time of peak HBsAg titer, suggesting that this enzyme is a manifestation of viremia and viral replication. DNA polymerase activity is usually transient but persist for years in chronic carriers and is an indication of continued infectivity.

In traditional Chinese medicine, the condition is thought to be caused by pathogenic damp-heat and patients with viral hepatitis may manifest different syndromes at different phases. It is usually divided into two types: Shaoyang disease and jaundice.

Shaoyang disease. The external affection at the stage between the exterior and interior parts of the body, with bitter taste in the mouth, dry throat, dizziness, intermittent fever, distress of the chest, restlessness, nausea, loss of appetite and stringy pulse.

Jaundice. Characterized by yellow-brown pigmentation of the skin and sclera and yellow coloured urine. It may be classified into two subtypes: constipation type and loose bowels type.

## CLINICAL MANIFESTATIONS

The clinical picture is extremely variable, ranging from asymptomatic infection without jaundice to a fulminating disease and death in a few days.

1. Prodromal phase. The speed of onset varies from abrupt to insidious, with general malaise, myalgia, arthralgia and occasionally arthritis, easy fatigability, upper respiratory symptoms (nasal discharge, pharyngitis), and severe anorexia out of proportion to the degree of illness. Nausea and vomiting are frequent and diarrhea or constipation may occur. Fever is generally present but is rarely over 39.5 degrees centigrade. Defervescence often coincides with the onset of jaundice. Chills or chilliness may mark an acute onset.

Abdominal pain is usually mild and constant in the upper right quadrant or right epigastrium and is often aggravated by jarring or exertion. On rare occasions, upper abdominal pain may be severe enough to stimulate cholecystitis or cholelithiasis. A distaste for smoking, paralleling anorexia, may occur early.

2. Icteric phase. Clinical jaundice occurs after 5 to 10 days but may appear at the same time as the initial symptomatology. Some patients never develop clinical icterus. With the onset of jaundice, there is often an intensification of the prodromal symptoms, followed by progressive clinical improvement.

3. Convalescent phase. There is an increasing sense of well-being, return of appetite and disappearance of jaundice, abdominal pain and tenderness and fatigability.

## DIAGNOSIS

Essentials of diagnosis in Western medicine.

• Anorexia, nausea, vomiting, malaise, symptoms of upper respiratory throat infection or "flu"-like syndrome, aversion to smoking.

• Fever, enlarged tender liver and jaundice.

• Normal to low white cell count; abnormal liver tests and liver function.

• Liver biopsy shows characteristic hepatocellular necrosis and mononuclear infiltrate.

In traditional Chinese medicine, the signs such as yellow-brown pigmentation of the skin and sclera and yellow coloured urine are also considered in making diagnosis.

## TREATMENT

**I. Treatment in Western medicine.**

A. General measures. Bed rest should be at the patient's option during the acute initial phase of the disease when the symptoms are most severe. Bed rest beyond the most acute phase is not warranted. However, return to normal activity during the convalescent period should be gradual. If nausea and vomiting are significant problems, or if oral intake is substantially decreased, the intravenous administration of 10% glucose solution is indicated. If the patient shows signs of impending coma, protein should be temporarily interdicted and gradually reintroduced and increased as clinical improvement takes place. In general, dietary management consists of giving palatable meals as tolerated, without overfeeding. Patients with infectious hepatitis should avoid strenuous physical exertion, alcohol, and hepatotoxic agents. While the administration of small doses of oxazepam or phenobarbital is safe (since they are not metabolized by the liver), it is recommended that morphine sulfate be avoided.

B. Corticotropin and corticosteroids. Although these agents have been recommended by some authors for the treatment of fulminant hepatitis, controlled studies have demonstrated no benefit in patients with severe viral hepatitis treated relatively early in the course of the disease.

## II. Treatment in Chinese medicine.

*1. Herb therapy*
For Shaoyang disease type.
Xiao Chai Hu Tang.
Constituents:

Chinese thorowax   24g
Skullcap  10g
Pinellia (tuber)  12g
Dangshen 15g
Winkled gianthyssop  12g
Shell of areca nut   15g
Dried old orange peel  12g
Fruit of hawthorn (baked)  30g
Medicated leaven (baked)   30g
Malt (baked)  30g
Capillary artemisia   60g·
Honeysuckle flower  30g
Weeping forsythia   30g
Loosestrife   60g

Decoction and dosage is the same.
For jaundice type with constipation.
Yin Chen Gao Tang Jia Jian.
Constituents:

Capillary artemisia    60g
Capejasmine  12g
Rhubarb  10g

Skullcap   10g
Chinese thorowax   12g
Honeysuckle flower   30g
Weeping forsythia   30g
Loosestrife   60g
Fruit of citron or trifoliate orange   12g
Fruit of hawthorn (baked)   30g
Medicated leaven   30g
Malt (baked)   30g

Decoction and dosage: All the above herbs make a dose and six to ten doses are prescribed with one dose daily. Each dose is simmered twice and then the broth of each mixed, half of the mixed broth each time, twice a day.

For jaundice type with loose bowels.

Yin Chen Shi Lin Tang Jia Jian.

Constituents:

Capillary artemisia   60g
Tuckahoe   30g
Umbellate pore   12g
Oriental water plantain   12g
Large-headed atractylodes   12g
Fruit of citron or trifoliate orange   12g
Fruit of hawthorn (baked)   30g
Medicated leaven (baked)   30g
Malt (baked)   30g
Loosestrife   60g
Asiatic plantain   30g
Cogongrass rhizome   60g
Honeysuckle flower   30g
Weeping forsythia   30g

Decoction and dosage is the same.

*2. Acupuncture therapy.*

Points: Sp9 Yinlingquan, S36 Zusanli, S9 Renying, B19 Danshu, B40 Yanggang and GV9 Zhiyang.

Method: All the above points are punctured with moderate stimulation and the needles are retained for 20 minutes. The therapy is given once daily.


# 6. CHRONIC HEPATITIS

## GENERAL CONSIDERATION

Chronic hepatitis is defined as a chronic inflammatory reaction of the liver with a duration of over 6 months as demonstrated by persistently abnormal liver tests. For proper treatment, it is crucial to determine whether the disease will resolve, remain static, or progress to cirrhosis. The causes of chronic hepatitis are only partially defined. It may be a sequela of infection resulting from hepatitis B virus. Chronic hepatitis has also been seen as a sequela of non-A, non-B hepatitis. Hepatitis A virus has not yet been shown to lead to chronic hepatitis. Additionally, identical clinical entitis may be associated with drug reactions, including oxyphenisatin, methyldopa and isoniazid.

### 1. Chronic persistent hepatitis

This form of chronic hepatitis represents an essentially benign condition with a good prognosis. The diagnosis is confirmed by liver biopsy. The biopsy may show portal tract infiltration with primarily mononuclear cells and occasional areas of focal inflammation in the parenchyma. The boundary between portal tracts and parenchyma remains sharp, and there is little or no "piecemeal necrosis." In essence, the architecture of the hepatic lobule remains intact. The symptomatology varies from the asymptomatic state to various vague manifestations including fatigability, anorexia, malaise and lassitude. Physical examination is usually normal.

Liver biopsy helps establish the diagnosis of persistent hepatitis. Treatment is mostly reassurance of the patient. Corticosteroids and immunosuppressive drugs should not be given. Dietary restrictions, excessive vitamin supplementation and prolonged bed rest are not necessary. The prognosis is excellent. Rarely does the disease progress to chronic active hepatitis.

### 2. Chronic active hepatitis

This form of chronic hepatitis is usually characterized by progression to cirrhosis, although milder cases may resolve spontaneously. The histologic changes include chronic inflammatory infiltration involving portal zones and extending into the parenchyma, with piecemeal necrosis and the formation of intralobular septa. Piecemeal necrosis, a process of inflammatory cells and hepatocyte necrosis occurring at the interface of the portal area and the liver lobule, may extend well into the lobule and across zonal boundaries. In severe cases, piecemeal necrosis may be associated with considerable hepatic failure or fibrosis and ultimately with cirrhosis. In very mild cases, it may be difficult to distinguish this entity from chronic persistent hepatitis. Liver biopsies repeated at varying intervals may be necessary to make the distinction as well as to monitor therapy.

The disease is thought to be caused by internal stasis of dampness and heat in traditional Chinese medicine. The pathologic changes due to damp and heat pathogens stay deeply in the body. Thereby, various manifestations of gastrosplenic and cholehepatic dysfunctions may occur.

## CLINICAL MANIFESTATIONS

### 1. Symptoms and signs

A. Chronic active hepatitis. This is generally a disease of young people, particularly young women. However, the disease can occur at any age. The onset is usually insidious, but about 25% of cases present as an acute attack of hepatitis. Although the serum bilirubin is usually increased. 20% of these patients have anicteric disease. Examination often reveals a healthy-appearing young woman with multiple spider nevi, cutaneous striae, acne and hirsutism. Amenorrhea may be a feature of this disease. Multisystem involvement, including kidney, joints, lung and bowel and coombspositive hemolytic anemia are associated with this clinical entity.

B. Chronic active hepatitis (HBsAg-positive type). This type of hepatitis clinically resembles the lupoid type of disease. The histologic pictures of these two types of chronic active hepatitis are indistinguishable. The HBsAg form of chronic active hepatitis appears to affect males predominantly. It may be noted as a continuum of acute hepatitis or may be manifested only by biochemical abnormalities of liver function.

*2. Laboratory findings*

The serum bilirubin is usually normal or only modestly increased (4.5-7mg/dL); SGOT (AST), IgG, IgM and gamma globulin levels are higher than normal. Late in the disease, serum albumin levels are usually decreased and prothrombin time may be significantly prolonged and will not respond to vitamin K therapy. Antinuclear and smooth muscle antibodies are positive 15-50% of the time. Latex fixation tests for rheumatoid arthritis and anticytoplasmic and immunofluorescent antimitochondrial antibodies are positive in 28-50% of patients. Hepatitis B antigen is not found in the blood of patients with classic "lupoid" hepatitis.

Activity in chronic liver disease can be defined quantitatively quite readily by establishing arbitrary biochemical standards. For example, either a 10-fold increase in serum transaminase level or a 5-fold elevation of SGOT with a 2-fold increase in gamma globulin concentration constitutes "high-grade" activity.

## DIAGNOSIS

Patients with chronic hepatitis may be entirely asymptomatic and exhibit only minimal abnormalities in routine laboratory tests, or may be incapacitated by progressive liver failure and the complications of portal hypertension. At any given time, the clinical and laboratory features may not correlate well with histopathology or long-term prognosis. For this reason and because concepts of the natural history and response to treatment are changing for some of these disorders, decisions regarding diagnosis, management and prognosis are often difficult and uncertain.

The concept of traditional Chinese medicine is that the stagnation of pathogenic damp and heat factors in the liver and the gallbladder influences and causes the spleen and stomach to become deficient. If this condition lasts for a long time, the stagnation of Qi and the depression of blood in the liver may occur.

## TREATMENT

### I. Treatment in Western medicine.

Prolonged or enforced bed rest has not shown to be beneficial. Activity should be modified according to the patient's symptoms. The diet should be well balanced without specific limitations other than sodium or protein restrictions as dictated by water retention or encephalopathy.

Prednisone has shown to decrease the serum bilirubin, SGOT and gamma globulin level and reduce the piecemeal necrosis in patients with chronic active hepatitis. Data from controlled clinical trials indicate that the mortality rate in the group of patients treated with corticosteroids is significantly reduced. However, relapse after discontinuation of prednisone therapy occurs frequently. In assessing the necessity for corticosteroid therapy, the benefit of the therapy should outweigh its potential risk. Patients with chronic active hepatitis who are symptomatic, those who are HBsAg-negative, and those who have severe histologic abnormalities appear at this time to be the most suitable conditions for corticosteroid therapy.

Prednisone or an equivalent drug is given initially in doses of 30mg orally daily, with gradual reduction to the lowest maintenance level (usually 15 to 20mg/dl) that will control the symptomatology and reduce the abnormal liver function. If symptoms are not controlled, azathioprine (Imuran), 50 to 150mg/d orally, is added with the primary benefit being that doses of corticosteroids can be much lower. Azathioprine imposes a significant hazard of bone marrow depression and complete blood counts should be obtained at least weekly or more frequently as dictated by the hematologic picture. In general, the combination of prednisone, 10 to 15mg/d, and azathioprine, 25 to 50mg/d, gives therapeutic efficacy with a paucity of significant side-effects of both drugs.

## II. Treatment in traditional Chinese medicine.

### 1. Herb therapy

For the type of liver stasis. Liver stasis is a short term for the stagnation and depression of the hepatic Qi. When the dispersing function of the liver is disturbed, there may appear various symptoms such as fullness or burning pain of the hypochondrium, chest distress, mental depression or anxiety, feeling of a lump in the throat, occasional epigastric distension and pain, hiccup, regurgitation of acid, suppressed appetite, occasional abdominal distension and pain, diarrhea. The treatment is to clear the liver with Xiao Yao San Jia Jian.

Constituents:

Root of Chinese angelica   20g
Unpeeled root of herbaceous peony  30g
Root of herbaceous peony   30g
Chinese thorowax   15g
Tuckahoe   10g
Large-headed atractylodes  15g
Nutgrass flatsedge   15g
Root-tuber of aromatic turmeric   12g
Rhizoma corydalis  12g
Fruit of hawthorn   15g
Medicated leaven   30g
Malt  30g
Capillary artemisia  30g
Loosestrife  30g

Decoction and dosage: All the above herbs make a dose and six to ten doses are prescribed with one dose daily. Each dose is simmered twice and then the broth of each mixed, half of the mixed broth each time, twice a day.

B. For the type due to the invasion of stomach by hepatic Qi. When the dispersing function of the liver is disturbed and the stomach is affected, there appear simultaneous pathologic manifestations of both the liver and the stomach. The main symptoms are vertigo, chest distress, hypochondriac pain, irritability and excitability, epigastric distension and pain, anorexia, nausea and vomiting, regurgitation of acid, stringy pulse, etc. The principle of treatment is to clear the liver and strengthen the spleen. The commonly used formula is Chai Ping Yin Jia Jian.

Constituents:

Chinese thorowax  12g
Pinellia   12g
Dangshen   12g
Skullcap  10g
Chinese atractylodes  12g
Bark of oficial magnolia  12g
Dried old orange peel  12g
Rhizoma corydalis  15g
Fruit of citron or trifoliate orange   15g
Fruit of hawthorn  10g
Medicated leaven  15g
Malt  30g
Capillary artemisia   30g
Loosestrife  30g

Decoction and dosage is the same.

C. For the type caused by depressed liver and insufficient spleen. When the dispersing function of the liver is disturbed and the spleen is affected, there appear simultaneously pathologic manifestations of the liver and the spleen. The main symptoms are vertigo, chest distress, hypochondriac pain, irritability and excitability, distension of the abdomen, loose stools, anorexia, stringy pulse, etc. The treatment is to strengthen the spleen and clear the liver with Qui Shao Liu Jun Zhi Tang Jia Jian.

Constituents:

Root of Chinese angelica   30g
Unpeeled root of herbaceous peony  30g
Root of herbaceous   30g
Dangshen  15g
Large-headed atractylodes (baked)  30g
Tuckahoe  15g
Dried old orange peel  12g
Pinellia  12g
Job's tears   30g
Chinese yan rhizome  30g
Fruit of hawthorn   30g
Medicated leaven   30g

Malt   30g
Winkled gianthyssop  12g
Capillary artemisia   30g
Loosestrife   45g

Decoction and dosage is the same.

D. For the type due to substantial heat in the liver and the gallbladder. The pathologic changes are due to stagnation of pathogenic damp and heat factors in the liver and the gallbladder. The main symptoms are jaundice, fever, bitter taste, pain in the hypochodrium, nausea and vomiting, anorexia, aversion to fatty food, abdominal distension and pain, yellowish urine, loose stools, yellowish glossy coating of the tongue, stringy and rapid pulse, etc. The treatment is to clear the heat and excrete the dampness with Yin Chen Shi Lin Tang Jia Jian.

Constituents:

Capillary artemisia  60g
Capejasmine  12g
Skullcap  10g
Loosestrife  60g
Tuckahoe  30g
Oriental water plantain  12g
Umbellate pore fungus  15g
Cogongrass rhizome  60g
Giant knotweed  30g
Fruit of hawthorn  12g
Medicated leaven 15g
Malt   15g
Rough gentian   15g

Decoction and dosage is the same.

E. For the type due to stagnation of Qi and blood. The liver is enlarged, palpable, firm if not hard, and has a blunt edge. The skin manifestations consist of spider nevi (only on the upper half of the body), palmar erythema (mottled redness of thenar and hypothenar eminences). The treatment is to break the stagnant Qi and activate the blood with Fu Yuan Hou Xue Tang Jia Jian.

Constituents:

Root of Chinese angelica  30g
Unpeeled root of herbaceous peony   30g
Chuanxiong  15g
Peach kernel  15g
Safflower  15g
Root of red rooted salvia  30g
Pangolinscale  10g
Rhubarb 6g
Chinese thorowax  12g
Nutgrass flatsedge  12g
Root-tuber of aromatic turmeric  12g

Zodoary turmeric 18g
Rhizoma corydalis 10g

Decoction and dosage is the same.

*2. Acupuncture therapy*

Points: B34 Yanglingquan, TE6 Zhigou and Liv14 Qimen.

Method: All the points are punctured with reducing method. But for patients with stagnation of Qi, B18 Ganshu and B40 Qiuxu are added to the prescription and for patients with stagnation of blood, B17 Geshu and Liv2 Xingjian are included.

3. Ear-acupuncture therapy.

Points: Chest Pt, Ear-shemen Pt and Liver Pt.

Method: Select 2 to 3 points on the affected side of the ear and puncture with the needles retained for 20 to 30 minutes.


# 7. CIRRHOSIS

## GENERAL CONSIDERATION

The concept of cirrhosis which evolved during the past few decades includes only those cases in which hepatocellular injury leads to both fibrosis and nodular regeneration throughout the liver. These features delineate cirrhosis as a serious and irreversible disease that is characterized not only by variable degrees of hepatic cell dysfunction but also by portosystemic shunting and portal hypertension. Fibrosis alone, regardless of its severity, is excluded by the previous definition, also excluded by definition are the earlier stages of chronic biliary obstruction and hemochromatosis, neither of which forms regenerating nodules until late.

An important part of this concept is the realization that the type of cirrhosis changes with the passage of time in any one patient. Terms such as "portal" and "postnecrotic" refer not so much to separate disease states with different causes as to stages in the evolution of cirrhosis.

Attempts to classify cirrhosis on the basis of cause or pathogenesis are usually unsuccessful when applied to individual patients. Such persons often represent end-stage cirrhosis, enabling only speculation about the evolutionary process. The use of purely anatomic and practical classification. One such classification that is currently employed divides cirrhosis into micronodular, mixed, and macronodular forms. It is important, however, to remember that these are stages of development rather than separate diseases.

A. Micronodular cirrhosis is the form in which the regenerating nodulars are no larger than the original lobules, i.e. approximately 1mm in diameter or less. It has been suggested that this feature results from the persistence of the offending agent (alcohol), a substance that prevents regenerative growth.

B. Macronodular cirrhosis is characterized by larger nodulars, which can measure several centimeters in diameter. This form corresponds more or less to postnecrotic cirrhosis but does not necessarily follow episodes of massive necrosis and stromal collapse.

C. Mixed macro- and micronodular cirrhosis points up the fact that the features of cirrhosis are highly variable and not always easy to classify. In any case, the configuration of the liver is determined by the mixture of liver cell death and regeneration as well as the deposition of fat, iron and fibrosis.

Finally, it should be emphasized that there does exist a limited relationship between anatomic types and etiology as well as between anatomic types and prognosis. For example, alcoholics who continue to drink tend to have that form of cirrhosis that remains micronodular for long periods. The presence of fatty micronodular cirrhosis, although not an infallible criterion, is strongly suggestive of chronic alcoholism. On the other hand, liver cell carcinoma not uncommonly arises in macronodular rather than micronodular cirrhosis. Although speculative and subject to dispute, it is possible that this propensity to malignancy is related either to the increased regeneration in macronodular cirrhosis or to the longer period required for the process to develop.

In traditional Chinese medicine, the condition is thought to be due to liver stasis or invasion of the stomach and spleen by hepatic Qi.

## CLINICAL MANIFESTATIONS

Micronodular cirrhosis may cause no symptoms for long periods both at onset and later in the course (compensated phase). The onset of symptoms may be insidious or less often, abrupt. Weakness, fatigability, and weight loss are common. In advanced cirrhosis, anorexia is usually present and may be extreme with associated nausea and occasional vomiting. Abdominal pain may be present and is related either to hepatic enlargement and stretching of Glisson's capsule or to the presence of ascites. Diarrhea is frequently present, but some patients are constipated. Menstrual abnormalities (usually amenorrhea), impotence, loss of libido, sterility, and painfully enlarged breasts in men (rare) may occur. Hematemesis is the presenting symptom in 15% to 25% of patients.

In 70% of cases, the liver is enlarged, palpable, firm if not hard, and has a blunt edge. Skin manifestations consist of spider nevi (usually only on the upper half of the body), palmar erythema (mottled redness of the thenar and hypothenar eminences), telangiectases of exposed areas, and evidence of vitamin deficiencies (glossitis and cheilosis). Weight loss, wasting and the appearance of chronic illness are present. Jaundice, usually not an initial sign, is mild at first, increasing in severity during the later stages of the disease. Ascites, pleural effusion, peripheral edema and purpuric lesions are late findings. The precoma state (asterixis, tremor, dysarthrias, delirium and drowsiness) and encephalopathy or coma also reflect the presence of alcoholic hepatitis. The superficial vein of the abdomen and thorax are dilated and reflect the intrahepatic obstruction to portal blood flow.

## DIAGNOSIS

Essentials of diagnosis.

● A past history of vital hepatitis, alcohol drink, schistosomiasis, deficient nutrition.

● The liver is enlarged, palpable, firm if not hard, and has a blunt edge.

● Blood chemical studies show primarily hepatocellular dysfunction, reflected by elevations of SGOT (AST), alkaline phosphatase and bilirubin. Serum albumin is low, whereas gamma globulin is increased.

● Liver biopsy shows cirrhosis.

● Symptoms and signs of portal hypertension.

## TREATMENT

### I. Treatment in Western medicine.

The principles of treatment include abstinence from alcohol and adequate rest, especially during the acute phase. The diet should be palátable with adequate calories and protein (75 to 100g/d) and in the stage of fluid retention. Sodium and fluid restriction. In the presence of hepatic precoma or coma, protein intake should be low or drastically reduced. Vitamin supplementation is desirable.

A. Ascites and edema due to sodium retention, hypoproteinemia and portal hypertension. Removal of ascites by paracentesis is usually not indicated unless it is critically important to relieve respiratory distress or patients discomfort or is essential for diagnosis of tumor or spontaneous bacterial peritonitis. Abdominal paracentesis can be associated with serious morbidity and even death. Hemorrhage, perforation of the bowel and abscess formation may occur.

In many patients, there is a rapid diminution of ascites on dietary sodium and fluid restriction alone. In individuals who pose more significant problems of fluid retention and who are considered to have "intractable" ascites, the urinary excretion of sodium is less than 10meq/L. Mechanisms that have been postulated to explain sodium retention in cirrhosis include impaired liver inactivation of aldosterone and increased aldosterone secretion secondary to increased renin production, which is associated with decreased renal cortical blood flow of uncertain causes. If such persons are permitted unrestricted fluids, serum sodium progressively falls, representing dilution, with a 200mg sodium diet and 500ml allowance of oral fluids per day, ascites production ceases and the patient's abdominal discomfort abates, however this regimen is unrealistic in most clinical situations.

a. Restoration of plasma proteins. This is dependent upon improving liver function and serves as a practical index of recovery. The use of salt-poor albumin intravenously is expensive, and the benefits are negligible.

b. Diuretics. Spironolactone should be used after documentation of secondary aldosteronism, as evidenced by markedly low urinary sodium. Starting with spironolactone, 50mg twice daily, and monitoring the aldosterone antagonist effect, reflected by the urinary sodium-potassium ratio and the fact that sodium excretion exceeds sodium intake. The dose of spironolactone is increased to 100mg every 3 days (up to a daily dosage of 1000mg) until the urinary sodium excretion exceeds 60meq/L. Diuresis commonly occurs at this point and may be augmented by the addition of a potent agent such as furosemide. This potent diuretic however, will maintain its effect even with a falling glomerular filtration rate, with resultant severe renal damage. The dose of furosemide range from 40 to 120mg/d, and the drug should be administered with careful monitoring of serum electrolytes.

The goal of weight loss in the nonedematous ascitic patient should be no more than 1 to 1.5 lbs/d.

B. Hepatic encephalopathy. Hepatic encephalopathy is the result if biochemical abnormalities associated with hepatocellular deficit or hepatic bypass of portal vein blood into the systemic circulation. Although disturbed ammonia metabolism is inherent in the clinical entity of hepatic encephalopathy, it is not clear that ammonia per se is responsible for the disturbed mental status. The amount of ammonia produced is dependent upon the protein content, the bacterial flora, the pH and the motility of the colon. Hepatic encephalopathy may also be further aggravated by the invasion of colonic organisms through the blood-stream. Bleeding into the intestinal tract from varices or ulcerations may significantly increase the amount of protein in the bowel and may precipitate rapid development of liver coma. Other factors that may precipitate hepatic encephalopathy include alkalosis, potassium deficiency induced by most diuretics, narcotics, hypnotics and sedatives; medications containing ammonium or amino compounds; paracentesis with attendant hypovolemia; and hepatic or systemic infection.

Dietary protein may be drastically curtailed or completely withheld for short periods during acute episodes. Parenteral nutrition is usually indicated.

Gastrointestinal bleeding should be treated by all necessary medical and surgical means to prevent further bleeding and to remove blood. Give milk of magnesia, 30ml 4 times daily, or magnesium sulfate 10 to 15g by indwelling nasogastric tube.

Lactulose (Cephulac), a nonabsorbable synthetic polysaccharide, acidifies the colon contents, resulting in retention of ammonium ion and decreased ammonia absorption. When given orally, the initial dose of lactulose for acute hepatic encephalopathy is 30ml 3 or 4 times daily, or a dose that will produce no more than 2 to 3 soft stools per day. The laxative effect is not beneficial in treatment. When rectal use is indicated because of the patient's inability to take medicines orally, the dose is 300ml of lactulose in 700ml of saline as a retention enema for 30 to 60 minutes; it may be repeated every 4 to 6 hours.

The intestinal flora may also be controlled with neomycin sulfate. 0.5 to 1g orally every 6 hours for 5 to 7 days. Side-effects of neomycin include diarrhea, malabsorption, superinfection, phototoxicity, otoxicity, and nephrotoxicity, usually only after prolonged use.

Treat infection with antibiotic agents chosen on the basis of culture and sensitivity studies. In some cases, broad-spectrum antimicrobials are indicated if the patient's condition is deteriorating.

If agitation is marked, give oxazepam, 10 to 30mg orally or sodium phenobarbital, 15 to 30mg intramuscularly, cautiously as indicated. Avoid narcotics, tranquilizers and sedatives excreted by the liver.

## II. Treatment in traditional Chinese medicine.

### 1. Herb therapy

A. For the type due to liver stasis. When the dispersing function of the liver is disturbed, there may appear various symptoms such as fullness or burning pain of the hypochondrium, chest distress, mental depression or anxiety, occasional epigastric distension and pain, hiccup, regurgitation of acid, suppressed appetite, occasional abdominal distension and pain, and diarrhea. The treatment is intended to clear the liver with Xiao Yao San Jia Jian.

Constituents:

Chinese angelica 20g
Unpeeled root of herbaceous peony 30g
Root of herbaceous peony 30g
Chinese thorowax 15g
Tuckahoe 10g
Large-headed atractylodes 15g
Nutgrass flatsedge 15g
Root-tuber of aromatic turmeris 12g
Rhizoma corydalis 12g
Fruit of hawthorn 15g
Medicated leaven 30g
Malt 30g
Capillary artemisia 30g
Loosestrife 30g
Root of red rooted saliva 30g
Zedoary turmeric 30g

Decoction and dosage: All the above herbs make a dose and six to ten doses are prescribed with one dose daily. Each dose is simmered twice and then the broth of each mixed, half of the mixed broth each time, twice a day.

B. For the type due to the stagnation of Qi and blood. The liver is enlarged, palpable, firm if not hard, and has a blunt edge, and the skin manifestations consist of spider nevi (usually only on the upper half of the body), palmar erythema (mottled redness of the thenar and hypothenar eminences). The treatment is to break the stagnant Qi and activate the blood with Fu Yuan Hao Xue Tang Jia Jian.

Constituents:

Chinese angelica 30g
Unpeeled root of herbaceous peony 30g
Chuangxiong 15g
Peach kernel 15g
Safflower 15g
Root of red rooted salvia 30g
Pangolinscale 10g
Rhubarb 6g
Chinese thorowax 12g
Nutgrass flatsedge 12g

Root-tuber of aromatic turmeris  12g
Zedoary turmeric  18g
Rhizoma corydalis  10g

Decoction and dosage is the same.

C. For the type due to splenic edema. Its chief symptoms are enlarged abdomen, edema and heaviness of the limbs, fatigue and shortness of breath, hydroperitoneum, generalized edema with abdominal distention, the pathologic changes due to the retention of water and dampness. As a result of the decline of the metabolic and transmissive function of the spleen, the main symptoms are anorexia, epigastric distress, abdominal distention, loose stools, nausea, no thirst or preference for hot drinks, general anasarca, lassitude and weakness, thick glossy coating of the tongue, slow and formicant pulse, etc. The treatment is to strengthen the spleen and excrete the dampness with Wu Lin San He Wu Pi Yin Jia Jian.

Constituents:

Tuckahoe peel  60g
Chinese waxgourd peel  60g
Scleratium  15g
Oriental water plantain  12g
Cassia  10g
Large-headed atractylodes  15g
Root-bark of white mulberry  20g
Shell of areca nut  15g
Seed of pepperweed or flixweed tansymustard  18g
Common reed rhizome  30g
Asiatic plantain  30g
Nutgrass flatsedge  15g
Root-tuber of aromatic turmeris  12g
Fruit of hawthorn  30g
Medicated leaven  30g
Malt (baked)  30g

Decoction and dosage is the same.

D. For the type due to the unconsciousness of the mind caused by heat and damp. The main symptoms are disorientation, coma or mental confusion, delirium, mania and excitability, jaundice, red tongue with yellowish and glossy coating, slippery and rapid pulse, etc. The treatment is to clear the heat and excrete the dampness for resuscitation with Yin Chen Gao Tang Jia Jian.

Constituents:

Capillary artemisia  60g
Capejasmine  12g
Rhubarb  10g
Loosestrife  60g
Giant knotweed  30g
Honeysuckle flower  30g
Weeping Forsythia  30g

Skullcap  10g
Chinese goldthread  10g
Buffalo horn  30g
Tabasheer  12g
Jack-in-the-pulpit  12g
Musk  0.06g

Decoction and dosage is the same.

# 8. CHOLECYSTITIS AND CHOLELITHIASIS

## GENERAL CONSIDERATION

Cholecystitis is associated with gallstones in over 90% of cases. It occurs when a calculus becomes impacted in the cystic duct and inflammation develops behind the obstruction. Vascular abnormalities of the bile or pancreatitis may rarely produce cholecystitis in the absence of gallstones. If the obstruction is not relieved, pressure builds up within the gallbladder as a result of continued secretion. Primarily as a result of ischemic changes secondary to distention, gangrene may develop with resulting perforation. Although generalized peritonitis is possible, the leak usually remains localized and forms a chronic, well-circumscribed abscess cavity.

Gallstones are more common in women than in men and increase in incidence in both sexes and all races with aging.

The simplest classification of gallstones is based on the chemical composition: stones containing predominantly cholesterol and stones containing predominantly calcium bilirubinate.

Three compounds comprise 80% to 95% of the total solids dissolved in bile; conjugated bile salts, lecithin and cholesterol. Cholesterol is a neutral sterol; lecithin is a phospholipid; and both are almost completely insoluble in water. However, bile salts are able to form multimolecular aggregates (micelles) that solubilize lecithin and cholesterol in an aqueous solution.

In traditional Chinese medicine, the disease is considered to be caused by substantial heat which has stagnated in the liver and the gallbladder for a long time. The long internal stagnation of heat and dampness damages the gallbladder and results in the disease.

## CLINICAL MANIFESTATIONS

The acute attack is often precipitated by a large or fatty meal and is character-ized by the relatively sudden appearance of severe, minimally fluctuating pain which is localized to the epigastrium or right hypochodrium and which in the uncomplicat-ed case may gradually subside over a period of 12 to 18 hours. Vomiting occurs in about 75% of patients and in half of instances affords variable relief. Right upper quadrant abdominal tenderness is almost always present and is usually associated with muscle guarding and rebound pain. Jaundice is present in about 25% of cases and, when persistent or severe, suggests the possibility of choledocholithiasis. Fever is usually present.

Cholelithiasis is frequently asymptomatic and is discovered fortuitously in the course of routine radio-graphic study, operation, or autopsy.

## DIAGNOSIS

Essentials of diagnosis of cholecystitis.
- Steady, severe pain and tenderness in the right hypochodrium or epigastrium.
- Nausea and vomiting.
- Jaundice.
- Fever and leukocytosis.

Essentials of diagnosis of cholelithiasis.
- Routine of radio-graphic examination.

Films of the abdomen may show gallstones in 15% of cases. 99mTC hepatobiliary imaging agents (iminodiacetic acid compounds), also known as HIDA scan, are useful in demonstrating an obstructed cystic duct.

The term for both cholecystitis and cholelithiasis is the same in traditional Chinese medicine, but more often it is called "pain of hypochondrium" or "pain of epigastrium" and "jaundice."

## TREATMENT

### I. Treatment in Western medicine.

Acute cholecystitis will usually subside on a conservative regimen (withholding of oral feedings, intravenous alimentation, analgesics and antibiotics if indicated). Cholecystectomy can be performed a few days after institution of hospitalization.

If conservative treatment has been elected, the patient (especially if diabetic or elderly) should be watched carefully for evidence of gangrene of the gallbladder or cholangitis.

Operation is mandatory when there is evidence of gangrene or perforation. Operation during the first 24 hours can be justified as a means of reducing overall morbidity in good-risk patients in whom the diagnosis is unequivocal. It is usually best to defer surgery, if possible, in the presence of acute pancreatitis, unless choledocholithiasis is suspected.

A. Medical treatment. During the acute period, the patient should be observed frequently, with careful abdominal examination and sequential determination of the white cell count several times a day. Analgesics such as pentazocine or meperidine should be used for pain control. Morphine derivatives in effective dose are known to produce spasm of the sphincter of oddi and may cause spurious elevations of serum amylase. Meperidine may have the same effects but to a much lesser degree. Appropriate antimicrobial agent should be employed in all but most mild and rapidly subsiding cases.

B. Surgical treatment. When surgery is elected for acute cholecystitis. Cholecystectomy is the procedure of choice. Cholangiography should be performed at the time of operation to ascertain the need for common duct exploration.

There is disagreement about the desirability of cholecystectomy in patients with "silent" gallstones, it is generally agreed that diabetic patients should undergo gallbladder removal to avoid complications. Operation is mandatory for symptomatic cholelithiasis.

## II. Treatment in traditional Chinese medicine.

### 1. Herb therapy

A. For the type due to the substantial heat in the liver and the gallbladder. The main symptoms are jaundice, fever, bitter tastes, pain in the hypochondrium, nausea and vomiting, anorexia, aversion to fatty food, abdominal distension and pain, yellowish urine, yellowish glossy coating of the tongue, stringy and rapid pulse, etc. The principle of treatment is to clear the pathogenic heat and excrete the dampness with Xiao Chai Hu Tang He Yin Cheng Gao Tang Jia Jian.

Constituents:

Chinese thorowax    24g
Pinellia    12g
Dangshen    12g
Skullcap    12g
Capillary artemisia    60g
Capejasmine    12g
Rhubarb    10g
Loosestrife    60g
Honeysuckle flower 30g
Fruit of weeping forsythia  30g
Rough gentian  15g

Decoction and dosage: All the above herbs make a dose and six to ten doses are prescribed with one dose daily. Each dose is simmered twice and then the broth of each mixed, half of the mixed broth each time, twice a day.

B. For the type due to the stagnation of Qi (vital energy). When the dispersing function of the liver is disturbed, there may appear various symptoms. Pain of the hypochondrium, epigastric distension and pain, regurgitation of acid, suppressed appetite, abdominal distension and pain. The treatment is to clear the liver and regulate the Qi with Xiao Yao San Jia Jian.

Constituents:

Chinese angelica  30g
Unpeeled root of herbaceus peony    30g
Root of herbaceus peony  30g
Chinese thorowax  12g
Large-headed atractylodes  15g
Nutgrass flatsedge  15g
Root-tuber of aromatic turmeric  15g
Fruit of citron or trifoliate orange  15g
Capillary artemisia  40g
Loosestrife  60g

Capejasmine   12g
Fruit of hawthorn (baked)   30g
Medicated leaven (baked)   30g
Malt (baked) 30g
Membrane of chicken gizzard   12g

Decoction and dosage is the same.

C. For the type due to the stasis of Qi. The chief manifestations of this type are spastic pain of hypochodrium and epigastrium, fever, mild jaundice, nausea, suppressed appetite, cold clammy limbs, constipation, yellowish urine. The treatment is to clear heat and excrete Qi. The formula commonly prescribed is Da Chai Hu Tang Jia Jian.

Constituents:

Chinese thorowax   12g
Rhubarb 10g
Fruit of immature citron or trifoliate orange   12g
Skullcap   12g
Pinellia   20g
Root of herbaceous peony   30g
Capillary artemisia   30g
Loosestrife   60g
Corydalis tuntschaninovii   10g
Chinaberry fruit   10g
Nutgrass flatsedge   15g
Olibanum 10g
Common myrrh tree  10g
Root-tuber of aromatic turmeric  15g

Decoction and dosage is the same.

*2. Acupuncture therapy*

Main points: S25 Tianshu and S36 Zusanli.

Auxiliary points: CV14 Guanyuan, B20 Pishu and S37 Shangjuxu.

Method: All the above main points and 1 or 2 of the auxiliary  points are punctured each time with moderate stimulation. The needles are retained for 20 minutes. Moxibustion with moxa stick is applied to CV8 Shenque and all the abdominal points. The therapy is given once daily.

*3. Ear acupuncture*

Points: Liver Pt, Gallbladder Pt, Stomach Pt, Spleen Pt, Endocrine Pt.

Method: All the points are punctured each time and the needles are retained for 60 minutes.

4. Point injection therapy.

Points: The same points are selected as in acupuncture therapy.

Drugs: Vitamin B1, Vitamin B12 and 5% Chinese angelica solution.

Method; Any one of the above drugs can be prescribed and 2 of each of the main and auxilliary points are injected with 0.5 millilitre in each. The therapy is given once daily.

# Chapter IV
# DISEASES OF THE URINARY TRACT

## 1. ACUTE GLOMERULONEPHRITIS

### GENERAL CONSIDERATION

Glomerulonephritis is a disease affecting both kidneys. In most cases, recovery from the acute stage is complete. However, progressive involvement may destroy renal tissue, in which case renal insufficiency results. Acute glomerulonephritis is most common in children 3 to 10 years of age. Although 5% or more of initial attacks occur in adults over age 50. By far the most common cause is an antecedent infection of the pharynx and tonsils or of the skin with group A B-hemolytic streptococci, certain strains of which are nephritogenic. In children under age 6, pyodema (impetigo) is the most common antecedent; in older children, skin infection is rare. Nephritogenic strains commonly encountered include, for the skin, M type 49, 2 and 55; for pharyngitis, type 12, 1 and 4, rarely, nephritis may follow infections due to pneumococci, staphylococci, some bacilli and viruses, or, plasmodium malariae and exposure to some drugs, including penicillins, sulfonamides, phenytoin, aminosalicylic acid and aminoglycoside antibiotics. Rhus dermatitis and reactions to venom or chemical agents may be associated with renal disease clinically indistinguishable from glomerulonephritis.

The pathogenesis of the glomerular lesion has been further elucidated by the use of new immunologic techniques (immunofluorescence) and electron microscopy. A likely sequela to infection by nephritogenic strains of B-hemolytic streptococci is injury to the mesangial cells in the intercapillary space. The glomerulus may then become more easily damaged by antigen-antibody complexes developing from the immune response to the streptococcal infection. The C3 component of complement is deposited in association with IgG (rarely IgA or IgM) or alone in a granular pattern on the epithelial side of the basement membrane and occasionally in subendothelial sites as well. Similar immune complex deposits in the glomeruli can often be demonstrated when the organ is other than streptococcal.

Gross examination of the involved kidney shows only punctate hemorrhages through the cortex. Microscopically, the primary alteration is in the glomeruli, which show proliferation and swelling of the mesangial and endothelial cells of the capillary tuft. The proliferation of capsular epithelium produces a thickened crescent about the tuft, and in the space between the capsule and the tuft there are collections of leukocytes, red cells and exudate. Edema of the interstitial tissue and cloudy swelling of the tubule epithelium are common. Immune complexes are demonstrable by means of immunofluorescence techniques. As the disease progresses, the kidney may enlarge. The typical histologic findings in glomerulitis are enlarging crescents that become hyalinized and converted into scar tissue and obstruct the circulation through the glomerulus. Degenerative changes occur in the tubules, with fatty degeneration and necrosis and ultimate scarring of the nephron. Arteriolar thickening and obliteration become prominent.

In traditional Chinese medicine, the condition is thought to be caused by deficiency of the functions of the spleen, lungs and kidneys. If any of the three organs is insufficient, fluid will be retained because body water can not be transformed into Qi.

## CLINICAL MANIFESTATIONS

Most patients have a fairly clear history of preceding streptococcal infection or exposure to a drug or other inciting agent. Usually the infection is a pharyngitis which has been sufficiently served to keep the patient away from school or work, but occasionally the infection lies elsewhere—for example, an otitis media, a leg ulcer, or a surgical wound. Sometimes the infection can only be demonstrated by a positive bacteriologic culture, or presumed from the finding of a raised anti-streptomycin O titer.

The patient has usually recovered from the initial infection when manifestations of nephritis appear, some 7 to 20 days after onset of the original infection. The most common presenting symptom is edema, noted particularly in the face on first arising, hematuria is also a common first symptom, usually the urine has a brown colour, but occasionally it is frankly blood-stained. Less commonly the patient complains of reduced urine output, or of bilateral dull loin pain, which is probably caused by stretching of the renal capsules.

It is important to note that the edema present at the onset of the disease is the result of reduced renal excretion of salt and water. In an adult of average size the presence of generalized edema implies a weight gain of at least 5 kg. At this stage patients have not lost enough protein in the urine to develop hypoalbuminemic edema (nephrotic syndrome), although this complication may develop later. Nor is there any good evidence for the earlier views that the edema of acute nephritis is caused either by increased capillary permeability or by heart failure.

Vague malaise, nausea and headache are common in acute nephritis, but fever is usual and patients do not usually feel really ill, although they are often distressed by the appearance of edema. In mild cases the patient may be quite asymptomatic; the disease may be picked up only by examining the urine of a person known to have had a recent streptococcal infection.

Physical examination usually shows generalized edema and mild hypertension of the order of 140 to 160 systolic, 90 to 110 diastolic. Very occasionally hypertension is severe with retinal hemorrhages and exudates, pepilledema or hypertensive encephalopathy. Fluid retention, if marked, may lead to the signs of congestive cardiac failure with cardiac enlargement and triple rhythm, venous engorgement, hepatic distention and gross pulmonary and systemic edema.

Urine output is usually reduced, although the reduction is often not noticed by the patient. Complete suppression of urine is rare, and indications vary with severe attack of nephritis; this complication may develop within a few days of the onset, or urine output may gradually fall to nothing over several weeks. As might be expected, fluid retention is particularly severe in such cases, and unless rigid restriction of sodium and water has been instituted early. Edema and hypertension are particularly marked. Unless renal function returns rapidly, the symptoms of renal failure eventually appear with nausea and vomiting, twitching and pruritus, acidotic respiration and progressive anemia.

## DIAGNOSIS

Essentials of differential diagnosis.
• History of preceding streptococcal or, rarely, other infection.
• Concurrent systemic vasculitis or hypersensitivity reaction.
• Malaise, headache, anorexia, low-grade fever.
• Mild generalized edema, mild hypertension, retinal hemorrhages.
• Gross hematuria, protein, red cell, casts, granular and hyaline casts, white cells and renal epithelial cells in urine.
• Evidence of impaired renal function, especially nitrogen retention.

## TREATMENT

### I. Treatment in Western medicine.

*1. Specific measures*

There is no specific treatment for edema. Eradication of B-hemolytic streptococi with penicillin or other antibiotic is desirable. Adrenocorticosteroids and corticotropin are no value and may be contraindicative because they increase protein catabolism, sodium retention and hypertension. Immunosuppressive and cytotoxic drugs have been ineffective in this form of nephritis.

*2. General measures*

In uncomplicated cases, treatment is symptomatic and designed to prevent overhydration and hypertension. Hospitalization is indicated if oliguria, nitrogen retention and hypertension are present. Bed rest is of great importance and should be continued until clinical signs abate. Blood pressure and blood urea nitrogen should be normal for more than 1 to 2 weeks before activity is resumed. A guide to duration of bed rest is the urine: when protein excretion has diminished to near normal and when white and epithelial cell excretion has decreased and stabilized, activity may be resumed on a graded basis. Excretion of protein and formed elements in the urine will increase with resumption of activity, but such increases should not be great. Erythrocytes may be excreted in large numbers for months and the rate of excretion is not a good criterion for evaluating convalescence.

In the presence of elevated urea nitrogen and oliguria, dietary protein restriction is indicated. If severe oliguria is present, no protein should be given. If no nitrogen retention is apparent, the diet may contain 0.5g of protein/kg ideal weight. Carbohydrates should be given liberally to provide calories and to reduce the catabolism of protein and prevent starvation ketosis with severe diguria. Potassium intoxication may occur, requiring dialysis.

Sodium restriction varies with the degree of oliguria. In severe cases no sodium should be allowed. As recovery progresses, sodium intake can be increased.

Fluid should be restricted in keeping with the ability of the kidney to excrete urine. If restriction is not indicated, fluid can be consumed as desired. Occasionally, when nausea and vomiting preclude oral consumption, fluids must be given intravenously in amounts depending upon the severity of the oliguria. Glucose must be given in sufficient quantities to spare protein and prevent ketosis.

If edema becomes severe, a trial of an oral diuretic such as furosemide is in order. Extreme fluid overload and oliguria may require dialysis.

If anemia becomes (hematocrit less than 30%) severe, blood transfusion in the form of packed red cells may be given.

## II. Treatment in traditional Chinese medicine.

*1. Herb therapy*
A. For Yang edema.
Yang edema is opposite to Yin edema, with heat manifestations caused by failure of the lungs to play a clearing and descending role. The clinical manifestations are mainly puffiness in the upper part of the body, particularly in the head and face, yellowish red skin, constipation, thirst and deep and frequent pulse. The treatment is intended to clear heat and excrete dampness with Yuan Pi Jia Shu Tang Jia Jian.

The constituents of the formula are:

Chinese ephedra    10g
Gypsum   30g
Weeping forsythia    30g
Honeysuckle flower    30g
Adsuki bean 30g
Oriental water plantain   15g
Motherwort   60g
Cogongrass rhizome    60g
Tuckahoe   30g
Stigma of corn   60g
Root-bark of white mulberry 30g
Asiatio plantain   30g

Decoction and dosage. All the above herbs are put together into a boiler to be simmered twice and then the broth of each mixed, half of the mixed broth each time, twice a day. Two to four doses are prescribed.

B. For Yin edema.
Yin edema is due to the disturbance of the function of the spleen and kidney which cannot eliminate and regulate body water. Clinically, edema first appear at the

lower limbs with pale or dusky skin, tastelessness, loose stools and deep retarded pulse. The rule of treatment is to warm the Yang principle and excrete dampness with Ji Shen Sheng Qi Wan Jia Jian.

The constituents of the formula are:

Tuckahoe 30g
Scleratium 15g
Large-headed atractylodes 30g
Cassia 15g
Ox-knee 15g
Asiatic plantain seed 30g
Prepared rhizome of rehmannia rhizoma 12g
Chinese yam rhizome 30g
Fruit of medicinal cornel 30g
Oriental water plantain 15g
Motherwort 60g
Cogongrass rhizome 60g
Herba Lycopi 12g
Root of red rooted salvia 40g
Milk veteh 60g

Decoction and dosage is the same.

*2. Acupuncture therapy*

Points for Yang edema: L7 Lieque, LI4 Hegu, LI6 Pianli, Sp9 Yinlingquan and B28 Pangguangshu.

Points for Yin edema: B20 Pishu, B23 Shenshu, CV6 Qihai, S36 Zusanli and B39 Weiyang.

Method: All the above points are prescribed for puncture and the needles are retained for 20 minutes.

*3. Moxibustion therapy*

Moxibustion can be applied to B20 Pishu and B23 Shenshu for Yin edema, and CV9 Shuifen and CV6 Qihai for Yang edema.

# 2. INFECTION OF THE URINARY TRACT

## GENERAL CONSIDERATION

The term urinary tract infection denotes a wide variety of clinical entities in which the common denominator is the presence of a significantly large number of microorganisms in any portion of the urinary tract. Microorganisms may be evident only in the urine (bacteriuria) or there may be evidence of infection of an organ —ureteritis, prostatitis, cystitis, pyelonephritis. At any given time, any one of these organs may be asymptomatic or symptomatic. Infection in any part of the urinary tract may spread to any other part of the tract.

Symptomatic urinary tract infection may be acute or chronic. The term relapse implies recurrence of infection with the same organism, while the term reinfection implies infection with another organism.

In traditional Chinese medicine, the condition is thought to be due to accumulation and stagnation of the pathogenic damp and heat factors in the urinary bladder. The main symptoms are frequency and urgency of urination, painful urination with scanty urine. It belongs to "lin symptom complex" (abnormalities of micturition) category.

## CLINICAL MANIFESTATIONS

### 1. Lower tract involvement

Burning pain on urination, often with turbid, foul-smelling, or dark urine, frequency, and suprapubic or lower abdominal discomfort. There are usually no positive physical findings unless the upper tract is involved also.

Microscopic examination of a properly collected urine specimen usually shows significant bacteriuria and pyuria and occasionally hematuria. Bacteriuria is confirmed by culture. Leukocytosis is rare unless the upper tract is also involved.

### 2. Acute pyelonephritis

Sudden rise of body temperature to 102 to 105 degrees fahrenheit, shaking chills, aching pain in one or both costovertebral areas or flanks, and symptoms of bladder inflammation. Physical examination reveals tenderness in the region of one or both kidneys; at times, a tender kidney may be detected by palpation. Laboratory tests show polymorphonuclear leukocytosis, and the urine is laden with leukocytes. Stain of the sediment reveals numerous bacteria, usually gram-negative bacilli, and culture confirms this. In a small proportion of cases, culture is also positive.

## DIAGNOSIS

• General symptoms and signs: sudden rise of body temperature to 39 degrees centigrade, chilliness, fever, headache, malaise, nausea and vomiting.

• Urinal tract infection symptoms and signs: costovertebral angle pain and tenderness, abdominal pain, frequency of urine, urodynia, dysuria and lower abdominal discomfort.

• Laboratory findings: significant bacteriuria, proteinuria, pyuria. The bacteria in the urine are often coated with immunoglobulin as revealed by immunofluorescence. Leukocytosis is common with a marked shift to the left. Blood culture is occasionally positive.

## TREATMENT

### I. Treatment in Western medicine.

#### 1. Specific measures

A. For the first attack of urinary infection, give sulfisoxazole or trisulfapyrimidines, 4g daily in divided doses by mouth for 3 to 7 days. Infections limited to the lower tract are sometimes eradicated if treated for just 1 to 3 days with ampicillin, 2 to 4g/d; amoxicillin 1 to 3g/d; or trimethoprim-sulfamethoxazole, one 80mg/400mg tablet 2 to 4 times daily. Oral cephalexin, 2 to 4g/d, or cephradine, 2 to 4g/d, may be equally effective. Maintain an alkaline urine pH. If symptoms have not improved and the urine has not cleared, shown by microscopy on the fourth day of treatment, re-examine the urine for possible resistant microorganisms. Follow-up at 3-6 weeks after treatment is stopped should demonstrate absence of bacteriuria; otherwise, retreat.

B. For recurrence of urinary tract infection, select an antimicrobial drug on the basis of antimicrobial susceptibility tests of cultured organisms. Give the drug for 10 to 14 days in doses sufficient to maintain high urine levels. Re-examine the urine 2 and 6 weeks after treatment is ceased.

C. For second recurrence or failure of bacteriuria, perform tests of renal function and excretory urograms and consider referral to urologist for a work-up for possible obstruction, reflux and localization of infection in the upper or lower tract. Men with recurrent urinary tract infection and probable prostatitis as a persistent focus often fail to be cured by 10 to 14 days of treatment in these patients. A 12 to 20 week trial of trimethoprim-sulfamethaxazole or ampicillin is indicated if the organism is susceptible to that drug mixture.

*2. General measures*

Forcing fluids may relieve signs and symptoms but should be limited to amounts that will avoid undue dilution of antimicrobials in the urine. Analgesics may be required briefly for pain. Metabolic abnormalities such as diabetes mellitus must be identified and treated.

## II. Treatment in Chinese medicine.

*1. Herb therapy*

A. For heat Lin. The main manifestations are oscillations between chills and fever, distention and pain of the hypogastrium, difficulty of urination, dark urine, burning pain of the urethra on micturition, rapid pulse and yellow coating of the tongue. The rule of the treatment is to dissipate heat and detoxify the body. The common formula is Xiao Chai Hu Tang He Ba Zheng San Jia Jian.

Constituents:

Chinese thorowax  30g
Skullcap  12g
Gypsum  40g
Herba polygoniaviculare  30g
Fringed pink  30g
Scleratium  15g
Asiatic plantain seed  30g
Talc  18g
Dandelion  30g
Chinese violet  30g
Corktree  10g
Henon bamboo leaf  10g
Oriental water plantain  12g

Decoction and dosage. All the above herbs are put together into a boiler to be simmered twice and then the broth of each mixed, half of the mixed broth each time, twice a day. Two to four doses are prescribed.

B. For bloody Lin.

It is manifested by hematuria with urethral pains and distention and pain of the hypogastrium, usually the patients with rapid pulse and yellow coating of the tongue. The treatment is to cool blood and detoxify the body with Xiao Gai Yin Zi Tang Jia Jian.

Constituents:

Field thistle  30g
Cattail pollen  12g
Node of lotus rhizome  30g
Talc  18g
Fresh or dried rehmannia  30g
Henon bamboo leaf  10g
Oriental arborvitae  12g
Chinese violet  30g
Dandelion  30g
Garden burnet (baked)  30g
Skullcap  15g
Honeysuckle flower  30g
Corktree  15g

Decoction and dosage is the same.

C. For consumptive Lin.

One of the Lin symptom complexes, which is chronic with exacerbation of symptoms after overwork. It is mainly manifested as dribbling of urine, vague pain of the genitalia after micturition, lassitude, lower backache, hot palms and soles, and refractory to treatment. When chronic, the patients have weak pulse, enlarged, swollen tongue with glossy coating. The treatment is intended to nourish the kidney and clear the heat with Zhi Bo Di Huang Tang Jia Jian.

Constituents:

Rhizome of wind-weed  12g
Corktree  12g
Prepared rhizome of rehmannia rhizoma  12g
Chinese yam rhizome  24g
Fruit of medicinal cornel  24g
Tuckahoe  30g
Oriental water plantain  15g
Root-bark of peony  12g
Dandelion  30g
Chinese violet  30g
Parastitic loranthus  30g
Radix phlomis  15g

Decoction and dosage is the same.

*2. Acupuncture therapy*

Main points: B23 Shenshu, B28 Pangguangshu, CV3 Zhongji and Sp6 Sanyin-jiao.

Auxiliary points: B32 Ciliao, CV4 Guanyuan, Sp9 Yinlingquan and Liv3 Tai-chong.

Method: Two or three of each of the main and auxiliary points are prescribed for puncture with moderate stimulation. The needles are retained for 20 minutes and the therapy is given once daily.

*3. Point injection therapy*

Points: B23 Shenshu, B28 Pangguangshu, CV4 Guanyuan, CV3 Zhongji and Sp6 Sanyinjiao.

Drugs: 5% of Chinese angelica solution and 10% figwort root solution.

Method: Either of the two drugs can be prescribed and two or three of the above points are injected with 0.5 to 1 millilitre of the solution in each. The therapy is given once daily and a course includes ten injections.


# 3. NEPHROLITHIASIS

## GENERAL CONSIDERATION

Approximately 90% of kidney stones are composed of calcium salts; nearly all rest are urate stones. Cystine stones are formed in patients with rare hereditary metabolic disorder, cystinurua, and xanthine stones in the still rare condition. In perhaps one-third to one-half of cases, stone formation is related either to increased excretion of calcium or uric acid or to persistent alterations in urinary acidity favoring precipitation of the normally dissolved amounts of these materials. In the remaining cases, alterations in the physicochemical characteristics of urine that favour crystallization presumably occur, but the nature of such changes and the identity of the factors concerned are yet unknown.

This disease is called "stone Lin," which is one of the Lin symptom complexes in traditional Chinese medicine.

## CLINICAL MANIFESTATIONS

Often a stone trapped in a calix or in the renal pelvis is asymptomatic. If a stone produces obstruction in a calix or at the ureteropelvic junction, dull flank pain or even colic may occur. Hematuria and symptoms of accompanying infection may be present. Flank tenderness and abdominal distention may be the only finding.

The urine may contain red cells, white cells and protein. X-ray examination will reveal radiation stone. Excretory and retrograde urograms help to delineate the site and degree of obstruction and to confirm the presence of nonopaque stones (uric acid).

## DIAGNOSIS

Essentials of diagnosis.

● Often asymptomatic.

● Symptoms of obstruction of calix or ureteropelvic junction with flank pain and colic.

● Hematuria.

● Nausea, vomiting, abdominal distention.

● Chills and fever and bladder irritability if infection is present.

## TREATMENT.

### I. Treatment in Western medicine.

Small stones may be passed out. They do no harm if infection is not present. Large stones may require surgical removal if obstruction is present or renal function threatened. Nephrectomy may be necessary.

### II. Treatment in traditional Chinese medicine.

*1. Herb therapy*

The most effective formula is Ba Zheng San Jia Jian. Its constituents are:

Fringed pink  30g
Herba polygoni aviculare 30g
Talc  18g
Oriental water plantain 15g
Asiatic plantain  30g
Loosestrife  60g
Climbing fern  12g
Membrane of chicken gizzard 10g
Chinese violet  30g
Corktree  10g
Herba pyrrosiae 30g
Henon bamboo leaf  10g
Fruit of citron or trifoliate orange 15g

Decoction and dosage. All the above herbs make a dose and six to ten doses are prescribed with one dose daily. Each dose is simmered twice and then the broth of each mixed, half of the mixed broth each time, twice a day.

*2. Acupuncture therapy*

Points: CV3 Zhongji, Sp6 Sanyinjiao, B39 Weiyang and Sp9 Yinlingquan.

Method: All the above points are prescribed for puncture with moderate stimulation and the needles are retained for 20 minutes.

# Chapter V
# BLOOD DISEASES

## 1. APLASTIC ANEMIA

### GENERAL CONSIDERATION

Aplastic anemia may occur at any age. Its incidence is approximately 4 per million population per year. It is characterized by pancytopenia or a selective depression of red cells, white cells or platelets. Number of toxins have been implicated including therapeutic agents, especially chloramphenical, phenylbutazone and mephenytoin; cytotoxic agents; irradiation; hepatitis virus; benzene; and some insecticides. In over half of cases, the cause is not known.

As the symptoms of general weakness is thought to be due to deficiency of the blood, the condition in traditional Chinese medicine is called blood deficiency.

### CLINICAL MANIFESTATIONS

Anemia may cause lassitude, pallor, fatigue, tachycardia, thrombocytopenia, purpura, bleeding, neutropenia and infections with high fever.

The red cell count may be below 1 million/ul. The cells are usually slightly macrocytic. The reticulocyte count is often low but may be normal or even slightly elevated. The white blood cell count may be less than 2000/ul and the platelet count less than 30,000/ul. The serum bilirubin is usually normal or low. Bone marrow is fatty with very few red and white cells and megakaryocytes. Hemosiderin is present.

Fixed tissue section made from the marrow aspirate or biopsy and stained with hematoxylin and eosin is best for demonstrating the characteristic architecture of an aplastic bone marrow; smears of the aspirate stained with Wright's stain are not adequate for diagnosis.

### DIAGNOSIS

Essentials of diagnosis in Western medicine.
- Lassitude, pallor, purpura and bleeding.
- Pancytopenia, fatty bone marrow.
- History of exposure to an offending drug or x-ray radiation.

In traditional Chinese medicine, the diagnosis is based mainly on symptoms such as pallor, palpitation, anxiety, dizziness, easy loss of memory, pale tongue, faint pulse, impaired vision, numbness of the limbs and pale nail-bed. The condition is classified into the category of deficiency of the cardiac and liver blood which finally influences the Yang and Yin of the kidney.

## TREATMENT

### I. Treatment in Western medicine.

*1. General measures*

A very thorough search for possible toxic agents must be made. All unnecessary medications must be discontinued. A detailed history of the patient's personal and work habits is essential. Patients should be specifically asked whether they have taken any agents for infection, arthritis or convulsions and whether they have been exposed to radiation. Even after a careful search, no cause can be found in approximately half of the patients.

*2. Marrow transplant*

This is the treatment of choice for patients under 50 with severe aplastic anemia (hemoglobin below 7g/dl) who have an HLA-compatible donor. Graft-versus-host disease remains a major problem. Bacterial and fungal infections are the common complications. Patients who have never been transfused do better (90% survival compared to 50% in the previously transfused group).

*3. Androgenic steriods*

When marrow transplant is not feasible, a trial of these agents is warranted, although their efficacy in acute aplastic anemia is in some doubt. It usually takes 2 to 3 months to see an effect, if any. The most commonly used agents are as follows:

A. Fluoxymesterone, 40 to 100mg daily orally (tablets, 2.5 and 10mg).

B. Oxymetholone. Two and a half mg/kg/d orally (tablets, 2.5, 5, 10, and 50mg).

C. Methandrostenolone. Forty to 100mg/d orally (tablets, 2.5 and 5mg).

D. Testosterone enanthate. Two hundred to 400mg/kg/d, twice weekly intramuscularly (100 and 200mg/ml).

E. Nandrolone decanoate. One and a half to 3mg/kg/wk intramuscularly (50/ml or 100mg/ml).

*4. Other agents*

Corticosteroids are of little value and are sometimes used for their stabilizing effect on capillary fragility in patients with severe thrombocytopenia.

Lithium carbonate, 300mg 3 times daily, may be tried in an effort to raise the granulocyte count.

*5. Transfusion*

Transfusions are best given in the form of packed red cells. The blood does not have to be from the same day's procurement, but the maximum benefit for the longest duration is derived if the blood is no more than a few days old. Some patients receive 5 or 6 units given over a couple of days, others prefer small but more frequent blood transfusions.

### II. Treatment in traditional Chinese medicine.

*Herb therapy.*

In traditional Chinese medicine, aplastic anemia is divided into three types:

A. Deficiency of the cardiac blood and the spleen. The chief symptoms are pallor, palpitation, anxiety, dizziness, easy loss of memory and other various hemorrhagic symptoms and signs such as anorexia, pale tongue, faint pulse, etc. The general rule of treatment for this type is to tonify the blood and the common formula is Gui Pi Tang Jia Jian.

The constituents of the formula are:

Chinese angelica  30g
Dangshen  15g
Large-headed atractylodes  15g
Milk veteh  12g
Polygala tenuifolia  12g
Apricot kernel (baked)  30g
Seed of oriental arborviate  30g
Fruit of Chinese magnolicavine  20g
Donkey-hide gelatin (melted) 15g
Yerbadetajo  20g
Root of pseudo-ginseng 1.5g
Licorice root  9g
Prepared rhizome of rehmannia rhizoma  15g

Decoction and dosage. All the above herbs are put together into a boiler to be simmered twice and then the broth of each mixed, half of the mixed broth each time, twice a day. Two to four doses are prescribed.

B. The impairment of the liver and the kidney. In this type of pathologic change, the Yin (vital essence) fluids of both the liver and the kidney are simultaneously impaired. The main symptoms are sallow complexion, numbness of the limbs, pale nail-bed, dizziness, feeling of distension of the head, blurred vision, insomnia, spermatorrhea, soreness of the waist and knees. The pulse may be stringy, faint and rapid, or faint and weak. The rule of treatment for this type is to nourish the liver and the kidney with Zuo Gui Yin Jia Jian.

The constituents of the formula are:

Prepared rhizome of rehmannia rhizoma  12g
Fresh or dried root of rehmannia  12g
Fruit of medicinal cornel  20g
Root-bark of peony  12g
Chinese yam rhizome  20g
Fruit of glossy privet  30g
Fruit of Chinese wolfberry  15g
Yerbadetajo  20g
Tuber of multiflower knotweed  15g
Donkey-hide gelatin (melted)  12g
Milk veteh  30g
Chinese angelica  15g
Root-bark of Chinese wolfberry  20g

Root of herbaceous peony 20g
Root of pseudo-ginseng  1.5g
Dangshen  12g

Decoction and dosage is the same as above.

C. Deficiency of kidney Yang. The pathologic manifestations are due to the impairment of the renal function with the accompanying cold syndrome. The main symptoms are chilliness, cold limbs, lumbago, spermatorrhea, premature ejaculation, impotence, frequency of nocturia, sallow complexion, numbness of limbs, pale nail-bed, dizziness, pale tongue, deep and formicant pulse. The rule of treatment is to tonify the Yang with You Gui Yin Jia Jian.

The constituents of the formula are:

Prepared rhizome of rehmannia rhizoma  15g
Fruit of Chinese wolfberry  15g
Donkey-hide gelatin  15g
Solomonseal  30g
Malaytea scurfpea  12g
Seed of Chinese dodder  30g
Longspur epimedium  30g
Chinese cynomorium  15g
Saline cistanche  12g
Glue of tortoise plastron 12g
Deerhorn glue 12g
Dangshen 12g
Chinese angelica 20g
Milk veteh 40g
Root of pseudo-ginseng  1.5g
Rumex madaio makino  6g
Radix polygoni multiflori  12g
Leatherleaf milletia  20g

Decoction and dosage is the same.


# 2. PAROXYSMAL NOCTURNAL HEMOGLOBINURIA

## GENERAL CONSIDERATION

Paroxysmal nocturnal hemoglobinuria is a rare chronic hemolytic anemia of variable severity, characterized by rather constant hemoglobinemia and hemosiderinuria and recurrent episodes of acute hemolysis with chills, fever, pain and hemoglobinuria.

The basic disorder is a membrane defect; hemolysis is produced by interaction between the abnormal cells and several factors present in normal serum; magnesium, properdin and complementlike components.

In traditional Chinese medicine, the disease is termed "deficiency of blood."

## CLINICAL MANIFESTATIONS

The disease is characterized by chronic hemolysis with hemoglobinemia and methemalbuminemia, usually increasing during sleep, regardless of the time when the patient sleeps. During the period of hemolysis sufficient to cause hemoglobinuria, the urine passed on arising is usually brown or reddish brown. Most patients usually have anemia and some patients may have jaundice. But a few patients never have hemoglobinuria and some may have hemoglobinuria after months and years. Spleen and liver may be slightly enlarged. White cell and platelet counts are often decreased and the reticulocyte count is increased. The bone marrow is usually hyperactive but may be hypoplastic. Aplastic anemia occasionally precedes the clinical development of this disorder.

The indirect serum bilirubin is elevated. Hemoglobinemia and methemalbuminemia are often present. Haptoglobins are absent. LDH is markedly elevated and the red cell acetylcholinesterase level is low. The intrinsic red cell defect is demonstrated by finding hemolysis on incubation of the patient's red cells in acidified normal serum (Ham test). The sucrose hemolysis ("sugar water") test can be used for screening. Hemoglobin electrophoresis and osmotic fragility are normal and the Coomb's test is negative.

## TREATMENT

### I. Treatment in Western medicine.

A. Transfusion. Transfusion of washed, normal red blood cells is needed during periods of severe anemia. Transfusion of whole blood should be avoided in most cases, because constituents of normal plasma as well as leukocytes may accelerate hemolysis.

B. Androgens. Administration of androgens such as fluoxymesterone, 20 to 30mg daily by mouth, may be beneficial by stimulating erythropoiesis.

C. Prednisone. Used in severely affected patients for a short period of time.

D. Administration of iron. For those who develop evidence of iron deficiency.

Folic acid, usually 5mg daily by mouth, is indicated to meet the increased folate requirement.

### II. Treatment in traditional Chinese medicine.

*Herb therapy*

The general rules of treatment in traditional Chinese medicine are to activate blood, clear pathogenic heat and eliminate the damp with Shi Wu Tang Jia Jian.

Constituents:

Chinese angelica  20g
Unpeeled root of herbaceus peony   30g
Chuanxiong  12g
Motherwort  30g
Capillary artemisia  30g
Bracken  30g

Selfheal   30g
Cogangrass rhizome   60g
Inkfish bone   15g
Milk veteh   30g
Horsetail   12g

Decoction and dosage is the same as above.


# 3. IDIOPATHIC (PRIMARY) THROMBOCYTOPENIC PURPURA

## GENERAL CONSIDERATION

Thrombocytopenia is the result of increased platelet destruction; the platelet count is closely related to the rate of destruction. Normal platelet survival is 8 to 10 days. But the survival is usually only 1 to 3 days in chronic idiopathic thrombocytopenic purpura and even less in the acute form. Most patients have increased levels of IgG on their platelets. Despite an apparent increase in number of megakaryocytes in the marrows, platelet production is usually not increased; antibodies may disturb megakaryocytic development and lead to ineffective production. The disorder may be postinfectious, e.g. following infectious mononucleosis or rubella; may be caused by isoimmunity; e.g. following transfusions or in the neonatal period; may develop into diseases with autoimmune manifestations; e.g. lupus erythematosus or lymphoproliferative disorders; or may follow the use of certain drugs, e.g. quinidine, quinine, thiazides, sulfonamides, phenylbutazone, acetazolamide, aminosalicylic acid, gold, heparin and others.

The spleen while not large, contributes to the thrombocytopenia in 2 ways: (1) it sequesters the subtly damaged platelets and (2) it manufactures some antibody.

Acute thrombocytopenic purpura is more common in children; 85% of patients are less than 8 years old. It usually remits spontaneously in 2 weeks to a few months. Chronic thrombocytopenic purpura may start at any age and is more common in females. At onset it cannot be distinguished from the acute form by laboratory test. There may be clinical remissions and exacerbation, but the platelet count is always low.

## CLINICAL MANIFESTATIONS

The onset may be sudden with petechiae, epistaxis, bleeding gums, vaginal bleeding, gastrointestinal bleeding or hematuria. In the chronic form, there may be a history of easy bruising and recurrent showers of petechiae, particularly in pressure areas. The spleen is not palpable.

Laboratory findings. The platelet count is below 100,000/ul and may be below 10,000/ul. Platelets may be absent on the peripheral blood smear. White cells are not affected. Anemia, if present, is secondary to blood loss.

The bone marrow megakaryocytes are increased in number but not surrounded by platelets; they are abnormal, with single nuclei, scant cytoplasm, and often vascuoles. The chief value of the marrow examination is to rule out leukemia and aplastic anemia.

The bleeding time is prolonged but PTT and PT are normal. Clot retraction is poor. Prothrombin consumption is decreased in severe cases. Capillary fragility (Rumpelleeds test) is greatly increased. An antinuclear antibody (ANA) test and a prothrombin time and PTT should be done to look for lupus erythematosus, which may present as purpura.

## DIAGNOSIS

Essentials of diagnosis in Western medicine.
- Petechiae, ecchymoses, epistaxis, easy bruising.
- No splenomegaly.
- Decreased platelet count, prolonged bleeding time, poor clot retraction.

In traditional Chinese medicine, the condition is termed "yin purpura" or "blood symptom complex."

## TREATMENT

### I. Treatment in Western medicine.

#### 1. General measures

Patients should avoid trauma, sports, elective surgery and tooth extraction. All unnecessary medications and exposure to potential toxins must be discontinued.

Children with mild purpura following viral infections do not require any therapy. They should be observed until petechiae disappear and the platelet count returns to normal.

#### 2. Corticosteriods

Corticosteroids are warranted in patients with moderately severe purpura of short duration, especially when there is bleeding from the gastrointestinal or genitourinary tract. Corticosteroids are also given to patients with purpura who have complications contraindicating surgery. Prednisolone 10 to 20mg 4 times daily, is usually required to control bleeding. The dosage is continued until the platelet count returns to normal, and then it is gradually decreased.

#### 3. Splenectomy

Splenectomy is indicated for all patients with well-documented thrombocytopenic purpura of more than 1 year's duration, for all patients with moderately severe purpura who have relapsed 2 to 3 times after corticosteroid therapy and for all patients with severe idiopathic thrombocytopenic purpura who do not respond to corticosteroids.

#### 4. Immunosuppressive therapy

In patients who do not respond to corticosteroids and in whom splenectomy has failed to raise the platelet count, either vincristine, 1.4mg/m2, or vinblastine, 7.5mg/m2, once weekly intravenously for 4 to 6 weeks, may raise the platelet count to acceptable levels without further maintenance therapy.

### II. Treatment in traditional Chinese medicine.

*Herb therapy*

A. For purpura due to deficiency of Qi and stagnant blood.

The skin of the patient with petechiae and ecchymoses is easy to bruise, particularly in the pressure areas. Usually, the patients may feel short of breath with low and weak voice, and pale complexion. The tongue is swollen and delicate and the pulse is weak and rapid. The rule of treatment is to tonify Qi and activate blood. The most effective formula is Huo Luo Xiao Lin Dan Jia Jian.

The constituents are:

Chinese angelica  20g
Root of red rooted salvia  30g
Olibanum  6g
Common myrrh tree  6g
Unpeeled root of herbaceus peony  30g
Root-bark of peony  30g
Milk veteh  60g
Asian puccoon   30g
Madder  15g
Node of lotus rhizome   15g
Donkey-hide gelatin (melted)  10g
Licorice root   6g
Root of pseudo-ginseng  3g

Decoction and dosage. All the above herbs are put together into a boiler to be simmered twice and then the broth of each mixed, half of the mixed broth each time, twice a day. Two to four doses are prescribed.

B. For purpura due to failure of the spleen to regulate the blood.

The skin of the patient with petechiae ecchymoses is easy to bruise, but usually is accompanied with gastrointestinal bleeding or hematuria, vaginal bleeding, sallow complexion, emaciation, weakness of the limbs, edema, thick glossy coating of the tongue, slow and formicant pulse. The treatment is intended to tonify the Qi and the blood with Gui Pi Tang Jia Jian, which is especially effective for purpura with vaginal bleeding.

The formula is composed of:

Dangshen  15g
Large-headed atractylodes  18g
Milk veteh  30g
Chinese angelica  30g
Fruit of medicinal cornel  30g
Yerbadetajo  30g
Fruit of glossy privet  30g
Donkey-hide gelatin (melted)  15g
Root of pseudo-ginseng  3g
Node of lotus rhizome  30g
Hyacinth bletilla  30g

Decoction and dosage is the same.

If the condition is accompanied with gastrointestinal bleeding, the following formula is prescribed.

Constituents:

Fresh or dried root of rhemannia    30g
Root of Zhejiang figwort    30g
Flower of Chinese scholar-tree (baked)    30g
Garden burnet (baked)    30g
Rhubarb (root)  12g
Limonium bicolor  30g
Acalypha australis  30g
Polygonum multiflorum    15g
Polygonum amplexicaule  15g

Decoction and dosage is the same.

If the patient is complicated with hematuria, the following formula is preferred.

Constituents:

Field thistle    30g
Cattail pollen    12g
Node of lotus rhizome    30g
Talc  18g
Chinese angelica  20g
Fresh or dried root of rehmannia    30g
Henon bamboo  10g
Cogangrass rhizome  60g
Yerbadetajo  30g
Capejasmine    12g
Corktree  12g

Decoction and dosage is the same.

The spontaneous and permanent recovery rate in childhood idiopathic thrombocytopenic purpura is 75% and in all adult cases is 25%. Chinese herbs are remarkably effective because corticosteroids cannot be used for a long period of time.

# Chapter VI
# ENDOCRINE DISEASES

## 1. HYPERTHYROIDISM

### GENERAL CONSIDERATION

Thyrotoxicosis is one of the most common endocrine disorders. Its higher incidence is in women between age 20 to 40. When associated with ocular signs or ocular disturbances and a diffuse goiter, it is called Graves' disease. Instead of a diffuse goiter, there may be a nodular toxic goiter, or all the metabolic features of thyrotoxicosis may occasionally be present without visible or palpable thyroid enlargement. The latter form is quite common in the elderly patients who may even lack some of the hypermetabolic signs ("apathetic" Graves' disease) but may present with a refractory cardiac illness. Lastly, a poor understood syndrome of marked eye signs, often without hypermetabolism, may precede, accompany or follow treatment of thyrotoxicosis, and has been termed exophthalmic Graves' disease, exophthalmic ophthalmoplegia and malignant (progressive) exophthalmos (infiltrative ophthalmopathy). It has been associated in some instances with the findings of high level of long-acting thyroid stimulator (LATS), a 7s gamma globulin of extrapituitary origin, although this factor may not be causally related to the disease. LATS is consistently found in the dermopathy ("pretibial myxedema") associated with Graves' disease. Other substances (e.g. LATS protector or human-specific thyroid stimulator) and evidence for altered cell-mediated immunity have recently been demonstrated in Graves' disease. Current thinking on the pathogenesis of Graves' disease involves the formation of autoantibodies that bind to the TSH receptor in thyroid cell membranes and stimulate the gland to hyperfunction. These thyroid-stimulating immunoglobulins (TSI) are demonstrable by special techniques in the plasma of most (but not all) patients with Graves' disease.

In traditional Chinese medicine, it is thought that emotional changes such as anger, anxiety, worry and apprehension may result in liver stasis with the symptoms such as fullness or burning pain of the hypochondrium, chest distress, mental depression or anxiety, feeling of a lump in the throat etc. So the diagnosis of thyrotoxicosis in traditional Chinese medicine is "flaming of the liver fire" due to the invasion of the spleen by hepatic Qi.

## CLINICAL MANIFESTATIONS

Restlessness, nervousness, irritability, easy fatigability, especially toward the latter part of the day, and unexplained weight loss in spite of ravenous appetite are often the early features. There is usually excessive sweating and heat intolerance and quick movements with incoordination varying from fine tremulousness to gross tremor. Less commonly, patients' primary complaints are difficulty in focusing their eyes, pressure from the goiter, diarrhea or rapid, irregular heat action.

The patient is quick in all motions, including speech. The skin is warm and moist and the hands tremble. A diffuse or nodular goiter may be seen or felt with a thrill or bruit over it. The eyes appear bright, there may be a stare at times periorbital edema, and commonly lid lag, lack of accommodation, exophthalmos and even diplopia. The hair and skin are thin and of silky texture. At times there is increased pigmentation of the skin, but vitiligo may also occur. Spider angiomas and gynecomastia are common. Cardiovascular manifestations vary from tachycardia, especially during sleep, to paroxysmal atrial fibrillation and congestive failure of the "high-output" type. At times a harsh pulmonary systolic murmur is heard. Lymphadenopathy and splenomegaly may be present. Wasting of muscle and bone are common features, especially in long-standing thyrotoxicosis. Rarely, one finds nausea, vomiting and even fever and jaundice. Mental changes are common, varying from mild exhilaration to delirium and exhaustion progressing to severe depression.

Associated with severe or malignant exophthalmos is at times a localized, bilateral, hard, nonpitting, symmetric swelling over the tibia and dorsum of the feet. At times there is clubbing and swelling of the finger. It often subsides spontaneously.

Thyroid "storm," rarely seen today, is an extreme form of thyrotoxicosis that may occur after stress, iodine refractoriness, or thyroid surgery and is manifested by marked delirium, severe tachycardia, vomiting, diarrhea, dehydration, and, in many cases, very high fever. The mortality rate is high.

The T4 level and radioiodine and T3 resin uptakes are increased. On rare occasions, the T4 level may be normal but serum T3 elevated. The radioiodine uptakes cannot be suppressed by T3 administration. In toxic nodular goiter, a high radioiodine uptake in the nodule may be diagnostic if combined with elevated T4 or T3 and low TSH level. Serum cholesterol determinations are low, postprandial glycosuria is occasionally found. Urinary creatine is increased. Lymphocytosis is common. Urinary and, at time, serum calcium and phosphate are elevated. Serum alkaline phosphatase is often elevated. An elevated LATS (Long-acting thyroid stimulator) level, and thyroid-stimulating immunoglobulins (TSI) may be present in the serum of patients with Graves' disease. Antithyroid antibodies are often positive in Graves' disease. TSH is low and fails to rise after TRF administration.

## DIAGNOSIS

Essentials of diagnosis:
• Weakness, sweating, weight loss, nervousness, loose stools and heat intolerance.

- Tachycardia; warm, thin, soft, moist skin; exophthalmos; stare and tremor.
- Goiter, bruit.
- T4, radio-T3 resin uptake and radioiodine uptake elevated and the failure of suppression by T3 administration.

## TREATMENT

### I. Treatment in Western medicine.

Treatment is aimed at halting excessive secretion of the thyroid hormone. Several methods are available; the method of choice is still being debated and varies with different patients. The most widely accepted method in the past has been subtotal removal after adequate preparation. There is a greater tendency toward trying long-term medical treatment with antithyroid drugs to achieve remission of the disease and to use radioactive iodine therapy rather than surgical thyroidectomy for thyroid ablation except for large multinodular glands.

A. Subtotal thyroidectomy. Adequate preparation is of the utmost importance. One or two days are generally necessary for adequate preparation: one of the thiouracil group of drugs alone, or, preferably, a thiouracil plus iodine. The sympatholytic agent propranolol has been used successfully as the sole agent before surgery. This drug, however, does not return the patient to a normal metabolic rate, and most experts prefer to render the patient euthyroid prior to surgery.

a. Preparative use of thiouracil and similar drugs. Propylthiouracil has been most widely used and appears to be the least toxic. It is the thiouracil preparation of choice. The T4 invariably falls, the rate of fall depending upon the total quantity of previously manufactured hormone available from the gland or in the circulating blood. The average time required for the T4 to return to normal is about 4 to 6 weeks. If the drug is continued, the T4 will continue to fall until the patient becomes myxedematous.

The preparation is usually continued and surgery deferred until the T4 and T3 uptake are normal. There is no need to rush surgery and no danger of "escape" as with iodine. In severe cases, 100 to 200mg 4 times daily is generally adequate. Larger doses are occasionally necessary. In milder cases, 100mg 3 times daily is sufficient.

Propylthiouracil appears to be an ideal drug except for 2 disadvantages: the danger of toxic reactions and interference with surgery. Toxic reactions to propylthiouracil are rare, however. In practice, patients are instructed to watch for fever, sore throat or rash and to notify their physicians immediately if any of these occurs so that blood count and examination can be performed. If the white cell count falls below 3000/ul or if less than 45% granulocytes are present, therapy should be discontinued. Other rare reactions are drug fever, rash and jaundice. The second objection is of a technical nature; since the gland may remain hyperplastic and vascular, surgical removal is more difficult. For this reason, combined therapy, using propylthiouracil and iodine, is the method of choice in preparing patients for thyroidectomy.

Methimazol (Tapazole) has a mode of action similar to that of the thiouracils.

The average dose is 10 to 15mg every 8 hours. The smaller dosage is no guarantee against toxic reactions, especially skin rash, which are more common with this drug than with the thiouracils.

Carbimazole is rapidly converted to methimazole and is similar in action. The average dose is 10 to 15mg every 8 hours. Toxic side-effects are slightly more common with this drug.

b. Preoperative use of iodine. Iodine is given in daily dosage of 5 to 10 drops of strong iodine solution or saturated solution of potassium iodine with nonspecific therapy until the T4 has dropped toward normal. The sign and symptoms have become less marked and the patient has begun to gain weight. The disadvantages of preparation with iodine are that: (1) a few patients may not respond, especially those who may have received iodine recently; (2) Sensitivity to iodides may be present. (3) if there is too long a wait before surgery, the gland may "escape" and the patient may develop a more severe hyperthyroidism than before; and (4) it is generally impossible to reduce the T4 to normal with iodine alone.

c. Combined propylthiouracil-iodine therapy. The advantage of this method is that one obtains the complete inhibition of thyroid secretion with the involuting effect of iodine. This can be done in either of the following two ways:

Propylthiouracil followed by iodine appears at present to be the preoperative method of choice. The therapy is started with propylthiouracil about 10 to 21 days before surgery is contemplated and the iodine is continued for 1 week after surgery.

Concomitant administration of the 2 drugs from the start in dosages as for the individual drugs, i.e. 100 to 200mg propylthiouracil 4 times daily and strong iodine solution, 10 to 15 drops daily. This method is less commonly used and less desirable than sequential administration.

Patients who fail to be euthyroid after subtotal thyroidectomy can be retreated with propylthiouracil or with radioiodine.

d. Propranolol. This drug may be used alone for the preoperative preparation of the patient in doses of 80 to 240mg daily. It is the most rapid way of reversing some of the toxic manifestations of the disease, and less time is necessary to prepare the patient for thyroidectomy. It has been suggested as the treatment of choice for thyrotoxicosis in pregnancy. Since it does not reverse the hypermetabolic state itself, escape and even thyroid storm may occur in patients so prepared.

B. Continuous propylthiouracil therapy (medical treatment). Control of hyper-thyroidism with propylthiouracil alone is often the treatment of choice, especially in young people, who are not good candidates for $131_I$ therapy. The advantage is that it avoids the risks and postoperative complications of surgery, e.g. myxedema, hypoparathyroidism. The disadvantage is the remote possibility of toxic reactions plus the necessity of watching the patient carefully for signs of hypothyroidism. Since the advent of propylthiouracil, it appears that the incidence of toxic reactions is slight.

The drug is administered with 100 to 200mg every 6 to 8 hours and continued until the $T_4$ and $T_3$ uptake are normal and all signs and symptoms of the disease have subsided; then place the patient on a maintenance dose of 50 to 150mg daily, observing the thyroid function tests periodically to avoid hypothyroidism.

An alternative method is to continue with doses of 50 to 200mg every 6 to 8 hours until the patient becomes hypothroid and then maintain the $T_4$ at normal levels with thyroid hormone.

The duration of therapy and the recurrence rate with nonsurgical therapy have not been completely worked out. At present it would seem that of the patients kept on propylthiouracil between 18 and 24 months, about 50% to 70% will have no recurrence. Patients with large thyroid glands that fail to decrease in sign with medical therapy have a greater chance of recurrence of thyrotoxicosis after the cessation of therapy. In some laboratories, the levels of thyroid-stimulating immu-noglobulins have been helpful in predicting the outcome of medical therapy. Those having recurrences after cessation of treatment may be treated again with propyl-thiouracil, redioiodine or surgery.

C. Radioactive iodine ($131_I$). The administration of radioiodine has proved to be an excellent method for destruction of over-functioning thyroid tissue (either diffuse or toxic nodular goiter). The rationale of treatment is that the radioiodine, being concentrated in the thyroid, will destroy the cells that concentrate it. The only objections to date to radioiodine therapy are the possibility of carcinogenesis and the possibility of damage to the genetic pool of the individual treatment. Studies to date have failed to show evidence of these effects. Nevertheless, the use of radioiodine is generally limited to older age group; however, the age level is not absolute and some children may be best treated with radioiodine. Do not use this drug in pregnant women. A high incidence of hypothyroidism several years after this form of treat-ment has recently been recognized, but this has also been found in patients treated in other ways and may be the natural course of the disease. Prolonged follow-up, preferably with T4 and TSH measurements, is therefore mandatory. There is a greater tendency toward higher dosage redioiodine ablation of the toxic gland with subse-quent permanent replacement therapy with thyroid hormone, rather than using smaller doses initially, which may require retreatment and may still fail to prevent appearance of myxedema several years later.

D. Lithium. Lithium carbonate alone or as adjunct to radioiodine therapy has been investigated recently. The results are not promising.

## II. Treatment in traditional Chinese medicine.

### 1. Herb therapy

A. For liver stasis. When the dispersing function of the liver is disturbed, there may appear various symptoms such as fullness or burning pain of the hypochon-drium, mental depression or anxiety, feeling of a lump in the throat, occasional irregular menstruation, palpitation, dysphoria, insomnia, sweating, red tongue, faint and rapid pulse. The general rule of treatment of this type is to clear the liver and purge the fire with Dan Ge Xiao Yao San Jia Jian.

Constituents:

Root-bark of peony  12g

Capejasmine   12g

Chinese angelica   15g

Root of herbaceous peony   30g

Chinese thorowax   10g

Tuckahoe   10g

Large headed atractylodes   15g

Chuanxiong   12g

Fresh or dried root of rehmannia   15g

Root of Zhejiang figwort   15g

Chinese goldthread   10g

Fossil fragments   30g

Oyster   30g

Selfheal   30g

Decoction and dosage. All the above herbs are put together into a boiler to be simmered twice and then the broth of each mixed, half of the mixed broth each time, twice a day. Two to four doses are prescribed.

B. For hepatic fire. The main symptoms are headache, congestion of the eyes, distending pain of the eyes, irritability and restlessness, dysphoria, flushed face, palpitation, restlessness, anxiety, perspiration, red edge and tip of the tongue with yellowish coating, stringy and rapid pulse. The rule of treatment for this type is to dissipate heat and purge the liver fire with Long Dan Run Gan Tang Jia Jian.

Constituents:

Rough gentian   20g

Capejismine   20g

Skullcap   12g

Chinese thorowax   12g

Oriental water plantain   15g

Asiatic plantain seed   30g

Chinese angelica   20g

Fresh or dried root of rehmannia   20g

Fossil fragments   30g

Oyster   30g

Chinese goldthread   10g

Tuber of dwarf lilyturf   30g

Selfheal   30g

Decoction and dosage is the same.

*2. Acupuncture therapy*

Main points: P6 Neiguan, B20 Pishu, CV12 Zhongwan and S36 Zusanli.

Auxiliary points: B21 Weishu, H7 Shenmen and Sp6 Sanyinjiao.

Method: Each time two or three of each of the main and auxilliary points are punctured with weak or moderate stimulation. The needles are retained for 10 to 15 minutes and the therapy is given once daily. A course includes ten punctures.

# Chapter VII
# METABOLIC DISORDERS

## 1. DIABETES MELLITUS

### GENERAL CONSIDERATION

Clinical diabetes mellitus represents a syndrome with disordered metabolism and inappropriate hyperglycemia due to either an absolute deficiency of insulin secretion or a reduction in its biologic effectiveness or both. The national institutes of health in 1979 decided to defer a "functional" classification of diabetes that based upon insulin secretion characteristics or insulin sensitivity. It recommends classifying diabetes mellitus into 2 major types.

A. Type I. Insulin-Dependent Diabetes Mellitus (IDDM). This severe form is associated with ketosis in the untreated state. It occurs most commonly in juveniles but also occasionally in adults.

B. Type II. Non-Insulin-Dependent Diabetes Mellitus (NIDDM). This represents a heterogeneous group comprising milder forms of diabetes that occur predominantly in adults but occasionally in juveniles. Two subgroups of patients with Type II diabetes are currently distinguished by the absence or presence of obesity.

a. Nonobese NIDDM patients. These patients generally show an absent or blunted early phase of insulin release in response to glucose.

b. Obese NIDDM patients. This form of diabetes is secondary to extrapancreatic factors that produce insensitivity to endogenous insulin.

In traditional Chinese medicine, the modern term for the condition is "emaciation-thirst disease," but in ancient Chinese medicine, it is called "Shi Yi" or "Xiao Dan." The diagnosis is mainly based on symptoms such as thirst, polydipsia, polyphagia, emaciation and polyuria.

### CLINICAL MANIFESTATIONS

The classic symptoms of polyuria, thirst, recurrent blurred vision, paresthesias and fatigue are manifestations of hyperglycemia and thus are common to both major types of diabetes, likewise, pruritus vulvae and vaginitis are frequent initial complaints of adult females with hyperglycemia and glycosuria due to either absolute or relative deficiencies of insulin. Weight loss despite normal or increased appetite is a feature of IDDM, whereas weight loss is unusual in obese patients with NIDDM who have normal or increased levels of circulating insulin. These latter patients with the insulin-insensitive type of diabetes may be relatively asymptomatic and may be detected only after glycosuria or hyperglycemia is noted during a routine examination. Diabetes should be suspected in obese patients, in those with a positive family history of diabetes, in patients presenting with peripheral neuropathy and in women who have delivered large babies or had polyhydramnios, preeclampsia, or unexplained fetal losses.

## DIAGNOSIS

- The classic symptoms of polyuria, thirst, recurrent blurred vision, paresthesias and fatigue are manifestations of hyperglycemia.
- The fasting plasma glucose is over 140mg/dl on more than one occasion, further evaluation of the patient with a glucose challenge is unnecessary.
- Fasting plasma glucose is less than 140mg/dl in suspected cases. A standardized oral glucose tolerance test may be done.
- The National Diabetes Data Group recommends giving a 75-g glucose dose dissolved in 300ml of water for adults (1.75 per kg ideal body weight for children) after an over-night fast in subjects who have been receiving at least 150-200g of carbohydrate daily for 3 days before the test.
- Normal glucose tolerance is considered to be present when the 2-hour plasma glucose is less than 140mg/dl, with no value between zero time and 2 hours exceeding 200mg/dl. However, a diagnosis of diabetes mellitus requires plasma glucose levels to be 200mg/dl both at 2 hours and at least twice between zero time and 2 hours.
- Insulin levels during glucose tolerance test. Normal immunoreactive insulin levels range from less than 10 to 25μV/mL in the fasting state and 50 to 130μV/mL at 1 hour and usually return to levels below 100μV/mL by 2 hours. A value below 50μV/mL at 1 hour and less than 100 μV/mL at 2 hours in the presence of sustained hyperglycemia implicates insensitivity of B cells to glucose as the cause of hyperglycemia, whereas levels substantially above 100μV/mL at these times suggest tissue unresponsiveness to the action of insulin.

## TREATMENT
### I. Treatment in Western medicine.
A. Diet. Caloric restriction for obese patients and regular spaced feeding with a bedtime snack for patients receiving hypoglycemic agents, especially insulin.

A well-balanced, nutritious diet remains a fundamental element of therapy. However, in more than half of cases, diabetic patients fail to follow their diet. The reasons for this are varied and include unnecessary complexity of the prescription as well as lack of understanding of the goals by both the patient and the physician. In prescribing a diet, it is important to relate dietary objectives to the type of diabetes. In obese patients with mild hyperglycemia, the major goal of diet therapy is weight reduction by caloric restriction. Thus, there is less need for exchange lists. Emphasis on timing of meals, or periodic snacks, all of which are so essential in the treatment of insulinrequiring nonobese diabetics.

Because of the prevalence of the obese mild diabetic among the population of diabetics receiving therapy, this type of patient represents the most frequent and thus one of the most important challenges for the physician. Treatment requires an energetic, vigorous program directed by persons who are aware of the mechanisms by which weight reduction is known to effectively lower hyperglycemia and who are convinced of the profoundly beneficial effects of weight control on blood lipid levels as well as on hyperglycemia in obese diabetics. Weight reduction is an elusive goal that can only be achieved by close supervision of the obese patient.

B. Oral hypoglycemic drugs.

These are of 2 major types: Sulfonylureas and biguanides.

a. Sulfonylureas.

The mechanism of actions of the sulfonylureas when they are acutely adminis-tered is due to their insulinotropic effect on pancreatic B cells.

Tolbutamide (Orinase) is supplied in tablets of 500mg. It is rapidly oxidized in the liver to an inactive form and its approximate duration of effect is relatively short (6 to 10 hours). Some patients require only 1 to 2 tablets daily.

Acute toxic reactions are rare with skin rashes occurring infrequently. Prolonged hypoglycemia has been reported rarely.

Chlorpropamide (Diabinese) is supplied in tablets of 100 and 250mg. This drug, with a half-life of 32 hours, is slowly metabolized with approximately 20-30% excreted unchanged in the urine. The average maintenance dose is 250mg daily given as a single dose in the morning. Prolonged hypoglycemic reactions are more common than with tolbutamide, particularly in elderly patients, in whom chlorpropamide therapy should be monitored with special care. Doses in excess of 250mg or 375mg daily increase the risk of jaundice, which does not occur on the usual dose of 250mg/d or less.

Acetohexamide (Dymelor) is supplied in tablets of 250 and 500mg. Its duration of action is about 10 to 16 hours. Give 0.25 to 1.5g daily in one or 2 doses. Side-effects are similar to those of the other sulfonylurea drugs.

Tolazamide (Tolinase) is supplied in tablets of 100 and 250mg. Tolazamide is more slowly absorbed than the other sulfonylureas, with effects on blood glucose not appearing for several hours. Its duration of action may last up to 20 hours. If more than 500mg/d is required, the dose should be divided and given twice daily.

Glyburide (Micronase). Effective dosage varies from 2.5 to 20mg. Unfamiliarity with its great potency (100 times more potent than tolbutamide) may account for the recorded high incidence of severe hypoglycemic reaction, with occasional fatalities.

b. Biguanides.

In 1977, the US Department of Health, Education, and Welfare recommended discontinuing general use of phenformin (DBI. Meltrol), the only biguanide available in the USA. It was considered to be an imminent hazard to health because of its reported association with lactic acidosis. In many countries, however, phenformin and another biguanide, metformin, continue to be used, although in some of these the indications for biguanide therapy in diabetes are being re-evaluated.

Phenformin (DBI). Its duration of action may last up to 6 to 10 hours. It's supplied in tablets of 25mg. The initial dosage is 2 to 3 tablets daily, and then the dose is increased gradually according to the blood glucose and glycosuria. The daily dose is no more than 150mg.

Dimethylbiguanide (metformin) is supplied in tablets of 0.5g, 2 or 3 tablets daily.

C. Insulin is indicated for Type I (IDDM) diabetics as well as for nonobese type II diabetics with insulinopenia whose hyperglycemia does not respond to diet therapy either alone or combined with oral hypoglycemic drugs.

Insulin preparations—three principal types of insulin are available:

a. Short-acting, with rapid onset of action.

b. Intermediate-acting.

c. Long-acting, with slow onset of action.

Short acting insulin (unmodified insulin) is a crystalline zinc insulin provided in soluble form and thus is dispensed as a clear solution. All other commercial insulins have been specially modified to remain more prolonged action and are dispensed as turbid suspensions at neutral pH with either protamine in phosphate buffer (protamine zinc insulin and NpH) or varying concentrations of zinc in acetate buffer (ultralente and semilente). The use of protamine zinc insulin and semilente preparations is currently decreasing, and almost no indications for their use exist. Conventional insulin therapy can presently be accomplished with regular insulin dispensed in an infusion device or administered as multiple injections in association with any of 3 insulin suspensions (NpH, lente or ultralente) whose duration of action is prolonged.

Regular insulin (Regular Iletin I or II, Insulin injection, Actrapid, Velosulin) is a short-acting soluble crystalline zinc insulin whose effect appears within 15 minutes after subcutaneous injection and lasts 5 to 7 hours. It is the only type of insulin that can be administered intravenously or by infusion pumps. It is particularly useful in the treatment of diabetic ketoacidosis and when the insulin requirement is changing rapidly, such as after surgery or during acute infections.

Lente insulin is a mixture of 30% semilente with 70% ultralente insulin—Lente Iletin I or II (Eli Lilly), Monotard (NOVO), Lente Insulin (Squibb). Its onset of action is delayed, and because its duration of action often is less than 24 hours. Most patients require at least 2 injections daily to maintain a sustained insulin effect. Lente insulin has its peak effect in most patients between 8 to 12 hours, but individual variations in peak response time must be considered when interpreting unusual patients, while lente insulin is the most widely used of lente series, particularly in combination with regular insulin. There has recently been a resurgence of the use of ultralente in combination with multiple injections of regular insulin as a means of attempting optimal control in IDDM patients. Ultralente has a very slow onset of action with a prolonged duration, and its administration once or twice daily has been advocated to provide a basal level of insulin comparable to that achieved by basal endogenous secretion or the over-night infusion rate programmed into insulin pumps.

NpH (neutral protamine, hagedorn or isophane) insulin is an intermediate-acting insulin whose onset of action is delayed by combining 2 parts soluble crystalline zinc with 1 part protamine zinc insulin and protamine, so that neither is present in an uncomplexed form ("isophane").

The onset and duration of action of NpH insulin are comparable to those of lente insulin; it is usually mixed with regular insulin and given at least twice daily for insulin replacement in IDDM patients.

Mixtures of insulin--Since intermediate insulins require several hours to reach adequate therapeutic levels, their use in IDDM patients requires supplements of regular insulin preprandially. For convenience, these may be mixed together in the same syringe and injected subcutaneously in split dosage before breakfast and supper. When mixing insulin, it is necessary to inject into both bottles a quantity of air equivalent to the volume of insulin to be subsequently withdrawn. It is recommended that the regular insulin be withdrawn first, then the intermediate insulin. No attempt should be made to mix insulins in the syringe and the injection is preferably given immediately after loading the syringe.

Recently, Eli Lilly has expressed a preference for NpH over lente as being less likely to retard the rapid action of regular insulin when administered as a mixture to diabetic patients. They suggest that the excess zinc in lente insulin binds the soluble insulin and partially blunts its action, particularly when a relatively small proportion of regular insulin is mixed with lente. However, since complexes of protamine insulin could enhance the immunogenicity of insulin, the need to expose patients to an insulin preparation containing a second animal protein may lessen the advantage NpH has over lente despite its wider range of mixability with regular insulin. Questions concerning the proportions in which regular insulin can be mixed with NpH, lente, or ultralente insulin without affecting the rapidity of action of regular insulin and questions as to the differential immunogenicity of NpH versus lente insulin, are being currently investigated.

The patient requiring insulin therapy should be initially regulated under conditions of optimal diet and normal daily activities. In patients with IDDM, information and counseling should be provided about the advantages of taking multiple injections of insulin in conjunction with self blood glucose monitoring. If tight control is attempted, urine glucose measurements are not sufficient, and at least 3 measurements of capillary blood glucose are required daily to avoid frequent hypoglycemic reactions. A typical initial dose schedule in a 70kg patient taking 2200 kcal divided into 6 or 7 feedings might be 10 units of regular and 20 units of NPH insulin in the morning and 5 units of regular and 5 units of NPH insulin in the evening. The morning urine or capillary blood glucose (or both) gives a measure of the effectiveness of NPH insulin administered the previous evening; the noon urine or blood glucose reflects the effects of the morning regular insulin; and the 5:00PM and 9:00PM sugars represent the effects of the morning NPH and evening regular insulins, respectively. A properly educated patient might be taught to adjust insulin dosage by observing the pattern of glycemia and glycosuria and correlating it with the approximate duration of action and the time of peak effect after injection of the insulin preparations. Adjustments should be made gradually and preferably not more often than every 3 days if possible. There are no data available concerning the level of glucose control needed to avoid diabetic complications. A reasonable aim of therapy is to approach normal glycemic excursions without provoking severe or frequent hypoglycemia. What has been considered "acceptable" control includes blood glucose levels of 60 to 130mg/dl before meals and after an overnight fast and levels no higher than 180mg/dl 1 hour after meals and 140mg/dl 2 hours after meals. In patients with milder forms of insulinopenia who require insulin therapy, a single morning injection of a small dose of intermediate insulin may suffice to supplement their own endogenous insulin secretion.

## II. Treatment in traditional Chinese medicine.

### Herb therapy

In traditional Chinese medicine, the condition is divided into four types: emaciation of the upper part of the body, emaciation of the middle part of the body, emaciation of the lower part of the body and stagnant blood and Qi.

A. For emaciation of the upper part of the body. The chief symptoms of the type are polydipsia, slow pulse and white coating of the tongue. The treatment is to supply the body fluids and reinforce Qi with Zheng Yan Tang Jia Jian.

Constituents:

Root of Zhejiang figwort   30g
Fresh or dried root of rehmannia   30g
Tuber of dwarf lilyturf   30g
Dangshen   15g
Milk veteh   40g
Stem of noble dandrobium   15g
Root of Chinese trichosanthes   15g
Fruit of Chinese magnoliavine   15g
Smoked plum   10g
Chinese yam rhizome   30g
Fruit of medicinal cornel   30g
Root of kudzuvine   30g
Root of red rooted salvia   30g

Decoction and dosage. All the above herbs are put together into a boiler to be simmered twice and then the broth of each mixed, half of the mixed broth each time, twice a day. Two to four doses are prescribed.

B. For emaciation of the lower part of the body. The chief manifestation of this type is emaciation in spite of excessive appetite, accompanied by thirst and polyuria, substantive pulses and yellow coating of the tongue. The effective formula is Bai Hu Tang Jia Jian for producing body fluids with pungent-cold drugs.

Constituents of the formula:

Gypsum   30g
Root of red rooted saliva   30g

Tuber of dwarf lilyturb   30g
Fresh or dried root of rehmannia   30g
Root of Zhejiang figwort   30g
Stem of noble dendrobium   15g
Milk veteh   60g
Chinese yam rhizome   30g
Fruit of medicinal cornal   30g
Root of straight ladybell   15g
Prepared rhizome of rehmannia rhizome   30g
Drug solomonseal   15g
Root of kudzuvine   15g

Decoction and dosage is the same.

C. For emaciation of the lower part of body. The chief symptom is large amounts of milky urine accompanied by excessive thirst and drinking, with deep and rapid pulse and the black coating of the tongue. The formula for this type is Liu Wei Di Huang Tang Jia Jian.
Constituents:

Prepared rhizome of rehmannia rhizome   30g
Fruit of medicinal cornel   30g
Oriental water plantain   15g
Root-bark of peony   15g
Milk veteh   60g
Root of kudzuvine   15g
Root of red rooted salvia   30g
Fruit of glossy privet   30g
White mulberry fruit   30g
Fruit of Chinese wolfberry   15g
Chinese angelica   30g
Fruit of Chinese magnolivine   30g
Yerbadejo   30g

Decoction and dosage is the same.

D. For stagnant blood and Qi. The patient often feels pain in the precordial area, cold limbs, numbness of the limbs, loss or impairment of sensation of the limbs, retarded pulse and dark purple tongue or with tongue petechia, Tiao Heng Shi Wu Tang Jia Jian is prescribed.
Constituents:

Chinese angelica   30g
Unpeeled root of herbaceous peony   30g
Chuanxiong   30g
Fresh or dried root of rehmannia   30g
Prepared rhizome of rehmannia rhizoma   30g
Root of red rooted salvia   10g
Costusroot   10g
Motherwort   30g

Root of kudzuvine   20g
Peach kernel   12g
Safflower   12g
Ox-knee 15g

Decoction and dosage is the same.

Some herb pills are also very effective for the disease. The commonly prescribed pills are Yu Quan Pills and Xiao Ge Pills and Liu Wei Di Huang Pills.

# Chapter VIII
# JOINT DISEASES

## 1. RHEUMATIC FEVER

### GENERAL CONSIDERATION

Rheumatic fever is an uncommon, but by no means rare, delayed sequel of an upper respiratory tract infection caused by Group A hemolytic streptococci. The pathogenesis remains obscure. Multiple focal aseptic inflammatory lesions are the basis for the acute manifestations, which may include migratory arthritis, carditis, chorea, erythema marginatum and subcutaneous nodules. Recurrences of rheumatic fever are common following an untreated streptococcal infection in patients with a previous history of this disease. The acute disease is of limited duration, but the carditis may lead to permanent valvular damage. It is for this reason that extensive studies have been concerned with methods to prevent first attack as well as recurrences of rheumatic fever. Prevention can be achieved only by the prompt detection, diagnosis and treatment of streptococcal pharyngitis.

In traditional Chinese medicine, the condition is classified into external affections, caused by the six pathogenic factors, namely, wind, cold, summer-heat, dampness, dryness, fire and malignant infectious pathogenic factors.

### CLINICAL MANIFESTATIONS

#### 1. Carditis

Carditis is most apt to be evident in children and adolescents. In adults, it is often best detected by serial electrocardiographic study. Any of the following establishes.

A. Pericarditis. It is uncommon in adults and is at times diagnosed by the progressive increase in "heart shadow" on serial chest X-rays or by echocardiography.

B. Cardiac enlargement. Detected by physical signs or X-ray, indicating dilatation of a weakened, inflamed myocardium. Serial X-rays are often needed to detect the change in size.

C. Frank congestive failure. Right heart failure is more prominent in children, and painful liver engorgement is a valuable sign.

D. Mitral or aortic diastolic murmurs. Indicative of dilatation of a valve ring or the myocardium with or without associated valvulitis.

In the absence of any of the above definite signs, the diagnosis of carditis depends upon the following less specific abnormalities considered in relation to the total clinical picture.

a. Electrocardiographic changes. P-R prolongation greater than 0.04 second above the patient's normal condition is the most significant abnormality; changing contour of P waves or inversion of T waves is less specific.

b. Changing quality of heart sounds.

c. Pansystolic apical murmur that persists or becomes louder during the course of the disease and is transmitted into the axilla. The carey coombs short middiastolic murmur should be carefully sought.

d. Gallop rhythm. Difficult to differentiate from the physiologic third sound in children and adolescents.

e. Sinus tachycardia out of proportion to the degree of fever, persisting during sleep and markedly increased by slight activity.

f. Arrhythmias. Shifting pacemaker. Ectopic beats.

*2. Erythema annulare and subcutaneous nodules*

The former begins as rapidly enlarging macules that assume the shape of rings or crescents with clear centers.

The nodules may be few or many; are usually small (2cm or less in diameter), firm and nontender.

*3. Sydenham's chorea*

Sydenham's chorea may appear suddenly as an isolated entity. Eventually, 50% of cases have other signs of rheumatic fever. Girls are more frequently affected and occurrence in adults is rare. Chorea consists of continual, nonrepetitive, purposeless jerky movements of the limbs, trunk and facial muscles. Milder forms masquerade as undue restlessness as the patient attempts to convert uncontrolled movements into seemingly purposeful ones. These movements are made worse by emotional tension and disappear entirely during sleep. The episode lasts several weeks, occasionally months.

*4. Arthritis*

The arthritis of rheumatic fever is characteristically a migratory polyarthritis that involves the large joints squentially, one becoming hot, red, swollen and tender as the inflammation in the previously involved joint subsides. In adults, only a single or a small joint may be affected. The acute arthritis lasts 1 to 5 weeks and subsides without residual deformity—except for the rare persistent arthritis known as jaccoud's arthritis. Prompt response of arthritis to therapeutic doses of salicylates is characteristic (but not diagnostic) of rheumatic fever.

## DIAGNOSIS

Criteria for diagnosis.

A. Major criteria.

a. Carditis.

b. Sydenham's chorea.

c. Subcutaneous (fascial) nodules.

d. Erythema marginatum.

e. Polyarthritis.

B. Minor criteria.

a. Fever.

b. Polyarthralgia.

c. Prolongation of P-R interval.

d. Increased sedimentation rate.

e. Evidence of antecedent bata-hemolytic streptococcal infection.

f. Verified history of previous rheumatic fever or presence of rheumatic valvular disease.

The diagnosis of rheumatic fever is almost certain when 2 or more major criteria are present. Nevertheless, rheumatoid arthritis, neurocirculatory asthenia, infective endocarditis, connective tissue diseases, serum sickness, penicillin reaction and chronic infectious disease can reproduce the early manifestations of rheumatic fever.

Laboratory findings show a raised sedimentation rate or white cell count; a high or increasing titer of antistreptolysin O demonstrating an antecedent beta-hemolytic streptococcal infection; and occasional proteinuria and microscopic hematuria.

## TREATMENT

### I. Treatment in Western medicine.

*1. General measures*

Bed rest should be enforced until all signs of active rheumatic fever have disappeared. The criteria for this are as follows: return of the temperature to normal with the patient at bed rest and without medications; normal sedimentation rate; normal resting pulse rate (under 100 in adults); return of ECG to normal or fixation of abnormalities. The patients may then be allowed up slowly, but several months should elapse before return to full activity unless the rheumatic fever was exceedingly mild. Maintain good nutrition.

*2. Medical measures*

A. The salicylates markedly reduce fever, relieve joint pain and may reduce joint swelling.

Sodium salicylate or aspirin is the most widely used of this group of drugs; aspirin must be used if the patient has evidence of cardiac failure. The salicylates should be used with antacids after meal or with milk to reduce gastric irritation. A usually satisfactory dose for children is 15 to 25 mg/kg given every 4 hours during the day for a week with the dose then decreased by half. Adults may require 0.6 to 0.9g every 4 hours during the day to allay symptoms and fever. Caution: never use sodium salicylate or sodium bicarbonate in patients with acute rheumatic fever who have associated cardiac failure. Aspirin may be substituted for sodium salicylate with same dosages and precaution.

B. Penicillin should be employed in the treatment at any time during the course of the disease to eradicate any existing streptococcal infection.

C. Corticosteroids. There is no clear or consistent proof that cardiac damage is prevented or minimized by corticosteroids. Corticosteroids are effective anti-inflammatory agents for reversing the acute exudative phase of rheumatic fever and are probably more potent for this purpose than salicylates. A short course of corticosteroids usually causes rapid improvement in the acute manifestations of rheumatic fever and is indicated in severe cases. Give prednisone, 5 to 10mg orally every 6 hours for 3 weeks, and then gradually withdraw over a period of 3 weeks by reducing and then discontinuing first the nighttime, then the evening, and finally the daytime doses.

## II. Treatment in traditional Chinese medicine.

*Herb therapy*

A. For palpitation. Usually the palpitation is due to the insufficiency of cardiac Qi and is a decline of cardiac function. The chief symptoms are palpitation, shortness of breath, chest distress, perspiration, faint or irregular pulse. The treatment is intended to tonify the heart Qi and excrete dampness. The effective formula is Lin Gui Shu Gang Tang Jia Jian.

The constituents of the formula:

Tuckahoe   30g
Cassia   12g
Large-headed atractylodes   15g
Milk veteh   30g
Root-bark of white mulberry   30g
Shell of aveca nut   15g
Seed of peperweed or flixweed tansymustand   18g
Common reed rhizome   30g
Cortex acanthopancis   4g
Oriental water plantain   15g
Chinese angelica   15g
Motherwort   30g

Decoction and dosage. All the above herbs are put together into a boiler to be simmered twice and then the broth of each mixed, half of the mixed broth each time, twice a day. Two to four doses are prescribed.

B. For vascular Bi. Bi syndrome is mainly characterized by symptoms of the blood vessels. The chief manifestations are irregular fever, burning sensation of the skin, pain of the muscles the joints and erythematous rash and subcutaneous nodules. The treatment is to clear the heat and activate the blood. The formula prescribed is Yin Xiao San He Tiao Heng Shi Wu Tang Jia Jian.

The constituents of the formula are:

Honeysuckle flower  30g
Weeping forsythia (fruit)  30g
Jingjie  12g
Gypsum  60g
Cassia  12g

Chinese angelica    20g
Fresh and dried root of rehmannia    20g
Unpeeled root of herbaceous peony    30g
Root-bark of peony    12g
Chuanxiong    18g
Peach kernel    12g
Safflower    12g
Root of pseudo-ginseng    2g
Root of Zhejiang figwort    20g

Decoction and dosage is the same.

C. For Sydenham's chorea due to internal pathogenic wind. The chorea consists of continual nonrepetitive purposeless jerky movements of the limbs, trunk and facial muscles. Milder forms masquerade as undue restlessness as the patient attempts to convert uncontrolled movement into seemingly purposeful ones. The treatment is intended to calm the "wind" and activate the blood with Tiao Heng Shi Wu Tang Jia Jian.

The constituents are:

Fossil fragments    30g
Oyster    30g
Root of largeleaf gentian    12g
Root of ox-knee    15g
Preparared rhizome of rehmannia rhizome    15g
Chinese angelica    20g
Unpeeled root of herbaceous peony    30g
Chuanxiong    18g
Peach kernel    12g
Safflower    12g
Magnetite    20g
Parasitic loranthus    30g

Decoction and dosage is the same.

D. For heat Bi. It is usually caused by pathogenic heat factors and characterized by redness, swelling, heat and pain of the joints often with generalized heat manifestations, such as fever, chills, thirst, yellowish coating of the tongue, rapid pulse. The treatment is to clear the heat and activate the blood with Bai Hu Jia Gui Tang Jia Jian.

Constituents:

Gypsum    40g
Cassia    12g
White mulberry branch    30g
Parasitic loranthus    30g
Angelica    12g
Root of largeleaf    12g
Fangfeng    12g
Chinese angelica    20g

Chuanxiong   20g

Unpeeled root of herbaceous peony   30g

Common St. paulwort 30g

Ox-knee  15g

Decoction and dosage is the same.

# Chapter IX
# DISEASES OF GYNECOLOGY

## 1. DYSFUNCTIONAL UTERINE BLEEDING

### GENERAL CONSIDERATION

Abnormal uterine bleeding due to endocrine factors or a lack of responsiveness on the part of the endometrium to normal hormonal stimulation is common in females from the age of forty to fifty, and particularly in the years immediately preceding the cessation of menstrual periods. The same type of ovarian dysfunction is noted at the other end of the menstrual spectrum, during puberty and adolescence. There it is due to the immaturity of the ovary, in contrast to the older age group, in which either the aging ovary fails to respond in the usual way to normal or abnormal pituitary stimulation, or the target organ endometrium does not react consistently to the varying quantities of ovarian hormones. The defect is usually on the progestin side, and the cycles tend to be anovulatory. Before the bleeding can be considered functional the physician must be convinced that no organic cause for the bleeding is present.

In traditional Chinese medicine, the condition is termed metrorrhagia, a collective term for profuse metrorrhagic and continuous uterine bleeding.

### CLINICAL MANIFESTATIONS

A large number of patients who have an abnormal bleeding pattern at the age of 40 to 50. The patient experiences nothing except the symptoms of anemia, which are noticeable only after the bleeding has continued for some days or weeks.

### DIAGNOSIS

Essentials of diagnosis.
- Uterine bleeding at the age of 40 to 50.
- No organic cause for the bleeding is present.

### TREATMENT

**I. Treatment in Western medicine.**

*1. Curettage and hysterectomy*

In this particular age group, there is far less indication for hormone therapy than in the earlier reproductive years when one should and can be conservative since the likelihood of cancer as the explanation of bleeding is more remote. When no visible or palpable pathologic change is evident, yet the patient bleeds abnormally, a curettage is the best form of therapy. If the uterine bleeding is purely functional, this frequently provides a cure. Whether or not a hysterectomy is performed at the time of curettage will depend on the physical findings, the interpretation of the histologic picture seen on frozen section of the endometrial tissue removed and the extent of the uterine bleeding, as indicated by the type and amount of flow and the degree of anemia produced. In many instances other factors, unrelated to the vaginal bleeding, influence the surgeon in the direction of hysterectomy, such as pelvic relaxation or associated abnormalities like fibroids or endometriosis, unsuspected until the patient was under anesthesia.

### 2. Hormone therapy

If the surgeon has carried out extensive diagnostic measures and has good reason to believe that no cancer is present, he may take a calculated risk and give the patient progesterone therapy. Since much of the time functional bleeding is anovulatory, the hormone deficiency likely is on the progestin side and is due to the unbalanced stimulation of estrin upon the endometrium. The basic aim in such therapy is to provide a medical curettage that produces a complete sloughing of the endometrium, rather than the patchy desquamation that occurs with anovulatory periods.

The dosage schedule varies with the individual uterine bleeding problem. If the bleeding is excessive and continues, an injection should be given immediately. Fifty milligrams of proluton intramuscularly for three days should stop the bleeding and produce complete withdrawal of bleeding three days later. This period of flow may be profuse, but it should terminate in about four days. If the patient still has a recognizable cycle, but simply bleeds excessively at the time of her period. Delalutin, 2cc, should be given as one injection beginning on the eighteenth day of a 28-day cycle, or proluton, 20mg, given as an intramuscular injection daily for 5 days, withdrawal of bleeding should occur approximately ten days after the Delalutin or four days after the last proluton injection.

If the patient continues to bleed or the same excessive bleeding occurs in subsequent cycles, hormone therapy should be abandoned and hysterestomy performed after a preliminary curettage.

## II. Treatment in traditional Chinese medicine.

### Herb therapy

A. For the type due to the deficiency of the cardiac blood and spleen. The chief symptoms of this type are pallor, palpitation, anxiety, dizziness, easy loss of memory, pale tongue and faint pulse. The treatment is to tonify Qi with Gui Pi Tang Jia Jian.

Constituents:

Milk veteh (baked with honey) 60g
Dangshen 12g
Large-headed atractylodes 15g
Chinese angelica 30g

Tuckahoe  12g
Root of the narrow-leaved polygala  12g
Seed of wild jujube (baked)  30g
Longan pulp  15g
Donkey-hide gelatin  15g
Hairyvein agrimony  30g
Flower of Chinese scholartree (baked)  30g
Garden burnet (baked)  30g
Yerbadetajo  30g
Root of pseudo-ginseng  3g

Decoction and dosage: All the above herbs make a dose and six to ten doses are prescribed with one dose daily. Each dose is simmered twice and then the broth of each mixed, half of the mixed broth each time, twice a day.

B. For the type due to the instability of the renal Qi. The pathological manifestations of this type are incontinence of urine, uterine bleeding, frequency of nocturia, persistent leukorrhea, lumbago, lassitude, dizziness, tinnitus, amnesia, pale tongue, deep and formicant pulse. The treatment is to stop bleeding through tonifying the kidney Qi with You Gui Ying Jia Jian.

Constituents:

Prepared rhizome of rehmannia rhizoma  15g
Chinese yam rhizome   30g
Fruit of medicinal cornel  30g
Fruit of Chinese wolfberry  15g
Bark of eucommia  15g
Seed of Chinese dodder  30g
Parasitic loranthus  30g
Fossil fragments  30g
Oyster  30g
Donkey-hide gelatin  15g
Hairyvein agrimony  30g
Deerhorn glue  12g
Inkfish bone  30g

Decoction and dosage is the same.

C. For the mixed type of the above two. This type illness is due to both deficiency of the cardiac blood and spleen and the instability of the renal Qi. The treatment is to tonify the spleen and kidney with Wu Zhi Yan Zhong Wan He Shen Yu Tang Jia Jian.

Constituents:

Seed of Chinese dodder  30g
Fruit of Chinese wolfberry  15g
Red raspberry  15g
Fruit of Chinese magnoliavine  15g
Fruit of medicinal cornel  30g
Prepared rhizome of rehmannia rhizoma  15g

Chinese angelica  15g
Milk veteh  60g
Large-headed atractylodes  15g
Solomonseal  30g
Donkey-hide gelatin  15g
hairyvein agrimony  30g
Root of pseudo-ginseng  3g
Root of herbaceous peony  30g

Decoction and dosage is the same.

# 2. LEUKORRHEA
## (Vaginitis)

### GENERAL CONSIDERATION

Leukorrhea is not a disease but the manifestation of ovulation or of a local or systemic disorder. It may occur at any age and affects almost all women at some time. The most common cause is infection of the lower reproduction tract; other causes are inflammation, estrogen or psychic stimulation, tumor and estrogen depletion.

Leukorrheic discharge is usually white because of the presence of exfoliated or inflammatory cells. The persistence of some vaginal mucus is normal. Nevertheless, when soiling of the clothing or distressing local symptoms occur, the discharge must be considered abnormal.

Excessive moisture may add to normal body odor and may be a source of self-consciousness. Frequent bathing and drying of the parts should suffice. In Contrast, a strongly offensive odor may be an indication of genital infection.

The disease is termed "Dai Xia" (vaginal discharge) in traditional Chinese medicine.

### CLINICAL MANIFESTATIONS

Vaginal discharge with or without discomfort may be associated with itching when urine contaminates the inflamed introitus. The patient may complain of pudendal irritation, proctitis, vaginismus and dyspareunia.

Inflammation or ulceration of the vulvovaginal surfaces or cervix and a copious, white or coloured, usually odorous, discharge are usually present.

### DIAGNOSIS

Cytologic study of a smear of vaginal secretion is indicated for all parous patients and others who are sexually active or whenever cancer is suspected. The same preparation can be stained to show trichomonads, candida, or other organisms. Motile trichomonads are often seen in freshly voided urine contaminated with leukorrheic discharge. If these organisms are noted in a catheterized specimen, urethral and bladder involvement by the flagellate is likely. Culture of the trichomonad is difficult but may be successful when trichosel medium is used.

Leukorrhea associated with positive serologic tests may be a result of syphilis; a positive complement fixation test suggests lymphogranuloma venereum.

Inspect a fresh wet preparation of the vaginal fluid first for motile trichomonas vaginalis. Look for heavy clouding of the spread and especially the covering of epithelial cells ("clue cells") by myriads of small bacteria; these will probably be chlamydia trachomatis or gardnerella (haemophilus) vaginalis, previously termed corynebacterium vaginale. Then add 5% potassium hydroxide to lake blood cells as an aid in visualization of candida hyphase and spores. Examination of a gram-stained smear may identify intracellular gram-negative diplococci, other predominant bacteria and helminths. If possible, culture the vaginal fluid anaerobically and aerobically to identify bacterial pathogens. Thioglycolate medium is most useful in the culture of Gardnerella organisms.

## TREATMENT

### I. Treatment in Western medicine.

*1. General measures*

Utilize internal menstrual tampons to reduce vulvar soiling, pruritus, and odor. Coitus should be avoided until a cure has been achieved. Trichomonal and candidal infections require treatment of the sexual partner also. Relapses are often reinfections. Re-treat both parties.

Antipruritic medications are disappointing unless an allergy is present.

*2. Specific measures*

A. For trichomonas vaginalis vaginitis.

Metronidazole. 2g in a single dose at bedtime. The physician should treat the sexual partner similarly during the same interval. Insist upon condom protection against reinfection during coitus until both partners are free of T vaginal organisms.

Aminocrine hydrochloride. Allantion and sulfanilimide creams used vaginally twice daily for 1 week are not as effective as metronidazole.

B. For candida albicans.

Discontinue oral contraception; substitute condom protection temporarily. Vaginal clotrimazole, one 100mg tablet or one applicatorful of miconazole nitrate 2% in an aqueous cream at bedtime for 7 nights, is effective for vaginal candidiasis.

C. For Gardnerella vaginalis and chlamydia trachomatis vaginitis.

Metronidazole, 2g orally at bedtime.

Tetracycline, 500mg orally 4 times daily for 5 days.

Sulfathiazole, sulfacetamide, and benzoylsulfanilamide in cream form (sultrin), 1 application daily for 10 days.

D. For atrophic (senile) vaginitis.

Diethylstilbestrol, 0.5mg vaginal suppository, 1 every third day for 3 weeks. Omit medication for 1 week; then resume cyclic therapy indefinitely unless contraindicated.

Dienestrol vaginal cream, one application for 1 week, then resume cyclic therapy.

Premarin, 0.625mg orally daily for 3 weeks each month. After 1 to 3 months of treatment, perform an endometrial biopsy to rule out carcinoma or atypical hyperplasia that could become cancerous.

E. For gonorrheal vaginitis.

Aqueous procain penicillin G, 4.8 million units injected.

### 3. Local measures

Occasional warm saline or acetic acid douches may be beneficial in the treatment of leukorrhea.

### 4. Surgical measures

Cauterization, cryosurgery, conization of cervix, incision of Skene's glands, or bartholinectomy may be required. Cervical, uterine, or tubal disease (tumors, infection) may necessitate laparotomy, irradiation, or other appropriate measures.

## II. Treatment in traditional Chinese medicine.

### 1. Herb therapy

A. For leukorrhea due to the loss of normal function of the spleen. The excessive thready discharge from the vagina is white and mucoid, like egg white because the pathologic changes due to abnormality of digestive and transporting functions of the spleen, so the symptoms are decreased appetite, abdominal distension, sallow complexion, emaciation, weakness of the limbs, and edema. The treatment is intended to strengthen the spleen and excrete the dampness with Wan Dai Tang Jia Jian.

Constituents:

Dangshen   12g
Largeheaded atractylodes   15g
Root of herbaceous peony   30g
Chinese yam rhizome   30g
Asiatic plantain seed   30g
Mustard ear   12g
Chinese thorowax   12g
Coix seed   30g
Deer horn   12g
Gibko-nut   15g
Fossil fragments   30g
Oyster   30g
Common cockscomb   12g

Decoction and dosage: Put all the above herbs together to be simmered twice, then the broth of each mixed, half of the mixed broth each time, twice a day.

B. For leukorrhea caused by substantial heat in the liver and the gallbladder. The main symptoms are yellowish mucoid thready discharge from the vagina with itching and stench, yellowish glossy coating of the tongue, stringy and rapid pulse. The treatment is to clear heat and excrete dampness. The most effective formula is Long Dan Zhong Gan Tang Jia Jian.

Constituents:

Rough gentian  15g
Capejasmine  12g
Skullcap  12g
Chinese thorowax  15g
Oriental water plantain  15g
Asiatic plantain seed  30g
Chinese angelica  20g
Fresh or dried root of rehmannia  20g
Corktree  12g
Root of sophora flavescens  18g
Bark of tree of heaven  12g
Chinese violet  30g
Dandelion  30g
Shenchuangzi  12g

Decoction and dosage is the same.

*2. Acupuncture therapy.*

First prescription: CV4 Guanyuan, CV3 Zhongji, Sp6 Sanyinjiao, Sp9 Yinlingquan and G26 Daimai.

Second prescription: CV6 Qihai, CV2 Qugu, Sp6 Sanyinjiao, Sp8 Diji and G26 Daimai.

Method: The two groups of points are punctured alternately with moderate stimulation. The needles are retained for 20 minutes.

# 3. PREMENSTRUAL SYNDROME
## (Premenstrual Tension Syndrome)

### GENERAL CONSIDERATION

Premenstrual syndrome is a recurrent (monthly) variable cluster of troublesome symptoms and signs that develop during the 7 to 14 days before onset of menses. The disorder may be characterized by irritability, emotional liability, hypo- or hyperreactivity, headache, palpitations, cyclic acneiform rash, mastalgia and edema of the extremities. Manifestations subside when menstruation occurs. Emotional nulliparous women 30 to 40 years of age are most commonly affected. Cyclic physiologic disturbances account for the symptoms. Recent studies suggest that renin augmentation of the latter portion of the menstrual cycle activates the angiotensin system, resulting in release of norepinephrine and aldosterone. Premenstrual syndrome is believed to be a result of the action of increased biogenic amines and fluid and electrolyte disturbances. Prostaglandin may be responsible for the troublesome effects.

No gross endocrine or other physical dysfunction distinguishes the patient with premenstrual tension syndrome. Brief elevated serum prolactin has been reported in some patients.

Dread of an impending period or concern regarding pregnancy, elimination and femininity often are related concerns. Atypical pelvic pain and primary dysmenorrhea may be the associated problems.

In traditional Chinese medicine, the disease is called "Di Shar Mong," due to hepatic Qi or liver stasis.

## CLINICAL MANIFESTATIONS

Anxiety, agitation, insomnia, inability to concentrate, and a feeling of inadequacy are reported. Patients complain of mastalgia, nausea and vomiting, and diarrhea or constipation. Depression may colour the woman's affect, or she may be contentious and aggressive. Peculiar drives or unusual appetites are commonplace.

The emotional build-up parallels weight gain (edema) of up to 3 or 4 kg. The general and pelvic examinations are not otherwise specific. A prompt weight loss by diuresis follows the onset of the period. Laboratory findings such as serum prolactin may be elevated.

## DIAGNOSIS

- Emotional nulliparous women 30 to 40 years of age.
- Recurrent variable cluster of troublesome symptoms and signs that develop during the 7 to 14 days before onset of menses.
- Brief elevated serum prolactin has been reported in some patients.

## TREATMENT

### I. Treatment in Western medicine.

Sympathetic understanding, reassurance, simple analgesics, thiazide diuretics, judicious use of sedatives, sodium restriction and support stockings may provide relief for many patients with premenstrual syndrome. Psychotherapy alone is relatively ineffective. Behavior modification is sometimes of value in treating patients whose mothers have had a similar illness pattern.

Suppression of ovulation by oral contraceptive may give relief. High doses of progestins are sometimes beneficial, but this therapy is not often practical. Prostaglandin drugs may give relief.

Spironolactone, an aldosterone blocking agent, 25mg orally 2 times daily for 7 to 10 days prior to and through the menses, has been reported to be effective and well tolerated. Other diuretics and potassium supplements must be avoided with spironolactone administration.

### II. Treatment in traditional Chinese medicine.

#### 1. Herb therapy

For "liver stasis." There may appear various symptoms, such as fullness or burning pain of the hypochondrium, chest distress, mental depression or anxiety, feeling a lump in the throat, occasional epigastric distension and pain, hiccup regurgitation of acid, suppressed appetite, occasional abdominal distension and pain, diarrhea, stringy pulse. The principle of the treatment is to clear the liver with Dan Ge Xiao Yao San Jia Jian.

Constituents:

Chinese angelica   20g
Root of herbaceous peony   30g
Chinese thorowax   10g
Tuckahoe   12g
Large-headed atractylodes   15g
Nutgrass plagsedge   15g
Root-tuber of aromatic turmeric   12g
Root-bark of peony   15g
Capejasmine   15g
Fruit of citron or trifoliate orange   15g
Fruit of harwthorn   15g
Medicated leaven   15g
Malt   30g

Decoction and dosage: All the above herbs make a dose and six to ten doses are prescribed with one dose daily. Each dose is simmered twice and then the broth of each mixed, half of the mixed broth each time, twice a day.

For hepatic fire. It is caused by disharmony of the hepatic Qi. The symptoms are irritability, fullness, distension and pain of the chest and hypochondrium, distension and pain of hypogastrium, breast pain, irregular menstruation, headache and dizziness, restlessness. In severe cases, mania may appear with stringy rapid and forceful pulse, redness of the tip and edges of the tongue with yellowish coating. The principle of the treatment is to purge the live fire with Lun Dan Xie Gan Tang Jia Jian.

Constituents:

Rough gentian   15g
Capejasmine   12g
Skullcap   12g
Chinese thorowax   15g
Oriental water plantain   15g
Chinese angelica   15g
Fresh and dried root of rehmannia   20g
Root-bark of peony   12g
Capejasmine   12g
Root of herbaceous peony   30g
Motherwort   20g
Fruit of glossy privet   30g

Decoction and dosage is the same.

For impairment of liver and kidney. The pathologic changes in which the Yin (vital essence) fluid of the body, liver and kidney are simultaneously impaired. The main symptoms are dizziness, feeling of distension of the head, blurred vision, tinnitus, hot palms and soles, insomnia, soreness of the waist and knee, breast pain, irritability, stringy, faint and rapid pulse, or faint and weak pulse. The principle of treatment is to nourish the Yin fluid with Yi Guan Jian Jia Jian.

Constituents:

Tuber of dwarf lilyturb    30g
Fresh or dried root of rehmannia    30g
Beishashen    15g
Chinese angelica    30g
Chinaberry fruit    12g
Fruit of Chinese wolfberry  15g
Root of Zhejiang figwort    20g
Root of herbaceous peony    30g
Chuanxiong  15g
Fruit of glossy privet    30g
Yerbadetajo    30g
Root-bark of peony    12g
Capejasmine    12g

Decoction and dosage is the same.
*2. Acupuncture therapy*
Main points: CV6 Qihai and Sp6 Sanyinjiao.
Auxiliary points: Sp10 Xuehai, P6 Neiguan and H7 Shenmen.
Method: All the above points are punctured moderately. The needles are retained for 20 minutes and the therapy is given once daily.

# Chapter X
# DERMATOPATHY

## 1. URTICARIA AND ANGIOEDEMA

### GENERAL CONSIDERATION

Urticaria can result from many different stimuli. The pathogenetic mechanism may be either immunologic or nonimmunologic. The most common immunologic mechanism is the type I hypersensitivity state mediated by IgE. Another immunologic mechanism involves the activation of the complement cascade which produces anaphylatoxins. These in turn can release histamine, whether the pathogenesis is allergic or nonallergic and the modulating factors affect mast cells and basophils to release mediators capable of producing urticarial lesions. These mediators include histamine, serotonin, kinins, slow-reacting substance of anaphylaxis, prostaglandins, acetylcholine, degradation products of fibrin and anaphylatoxins that increase vascular permeability, producing wheals. Intracellular levels of CAMP have a modulating role in the secretory release of histamine from mast cells and basophils.

In traditional Chinese medicine the condition is termed "Yin Zhen," "Feng Zhen Kuai," "Feng Tuan" and "Pei Lei," and is thought to be caused by wind cold and heat. As the cold pathogen invades the body surface, the defensive mechanism which is called Wei in traditional Chinese medicine, referring to the Yang principle for defense at the body surface, is damaged, unable to protect the body externally, and the nutrients which is called Yin, being the materialistic foundation for sweat, cannot support the body internally. Hence, Yin Zhen occurs.

### CLINICAL MANIFESTATIONS

Itching is the classic presenting symptom but may be absent in rare cases. Lesions are acute with pseudopods and intense sweating. The morphology of the lesions may vary over a period of minutes to hours. There may be involvement of the lips, tongue, eyelids, larynx, palms, soles and genitalia. Papular urticaria resulting from insect bites may persist for long periods and may occasionally be mistaken for lymphoma or leukemia cutis on the basis of histologic findings. A central punctum can usually be seen as with flea or gnat bites. Streaked urticarial lesions may be seen in acute allergic plant dermatitis, e.g. poison ivy, oak, or sumac.

In familial angioedema, there is generally a positive family history and the urticarial lesions may be massive. Death may occur from laryngeal obstruction.

## TREATMENT

### I. In Western medicine.

Systemic treatment. Look for and eliminate the causes if possible. The chief nonallergic causes are drugs, e.g. atropine, pilocarpine, morphine and codeine; arthropod bites, e.g. insect bites and bee stings (although the latter may cause anaphylaxis as well as angioedema); physical factors such as heat, cold, sunlight, injury and pressure; and presumably, neurogenic factors such as tension states and cholinergic urticaria induced by physical exercise, excitement, hot showers, etc.

Allergic causes may include penicillin reactions, inhalants such as feathers and animal danders, ingestion of shellfish or strawberries, injection of sera and vaccines as well as penicillin, external contactants including various chemicals and cosmetics, and infections such as viral hepatitis.

A few patients with chronic urticaria may respond to a salicylate- and tartrazine-free diet. Although salicylates are ubiquitous in nature, drugs and food are the most obvious sources.

Systemic treatment include antihistamines orally. Hydroxyzine, 10mg twice daily to 25mg 3 times daily, may be very useful. Cyproheptadine, 4mg 4 times daily, may work where hydroxyzine fails and is especially useful for cold urticaria. It may be necessary to give a burst of oral prednisone in a dose of 40mg daily for 10 days. Epinephrine 1:1000, a few minims given subcutaneously and sequentially, may be very useful.

For hereditary angioedema, methyltesterone buccal tablets, 10mg once or twice daily, may reduce the episodes. Danazol is effective for hereditary angioedema, but is expensive. Stanazolol is a cheaper anabolic agent and is effective. Lyophilized, partially purified CI-inhibitor concentrate in 5% dextrose, given intravenously in 10 to 45 minutes, may be lifesaving during an acute attack.

There is a continued search for effective treatment for chronic idiopathic urticaria. The combined use of $H_1$ and $H_2$ receptor blockers such as chlorpheniramine and cimetidine, has given inconsistent results. The rational for using ketotifen and terbutaline in combination is to increase CAMP level and thereby inhibits mast cell degranulation, however, efficacy requires confirmation.

When urticarial lesions persist indefinitely, biopsy is necessary to rule out vasculitis, and it may be desirable to determine the erythrocyte sedimentation rate, quantitative immunoglobulins, cryoglobulins, cryofibrinogens, antinuclear antibodies, total hemolytic complement and circulating immune complexes. Hepatitis B is one factor that may cause persisting lesions.

### II. In traditional Chinese medicine.

#### 1. Herb therapy

In traditional Chinese medicine, the disease is considered to be caused by wind, because the wind syndrome is usually characterized by "mobility," "change" and "abruptness." The lesions of the disease are acute with pseudopods and intense swelling. The morphology of the lesions may vary over a period of minutes to hours. There may be involvement of the lips, tongue, eyelids, larynx, palms, soles and genitalia. So it belongs to wind disease and is usually divided into two types.

A. Wind-and-cold type.

Patients with urticaria caused by both wind and cold is characterized by deficiency of the Yang, a pathologic phenomena in which the Yang principle becomes insubstantive and the cold manifestations such as chilliness, coldness of the limbs, and pale complexion are relatively predominant, with enlarged tongue and weak pulse.

The treatment of this type in traditional Chinese medicine is to tonify Qi (vital energy) and remove blood stasis with Shi Wu Tang Jia Jian.

Constituents:

Milk veteh    50g
Chinese angelica    30g
Unpeeled root of herbaceous peony    30g
Chuanxiong    20g
Prepared rhizome of rehmannia rhizone    15g
Jingjie    12g
Asian puccoon    30g
Broom cypress fruit    60g
Cassia bark    15g
Cicada slough    20g
Shechuangzi    12g
Root-bark of ditlany    12g

Decoction and dosage. All the above herbs are put together into a boiler to be simmered twice and then the broth of each mixed, half of the mixed broth each time, twice a day. Two to four doses are prescribed.

B. Wind-and-heat type.

If the illness is caused by wind and heat pathogens, the characteristics of the illness is the deficiency of the Yin, a general pathologic phenomena in which the Yin principle becomes insubstantive and the heat manifestations such as low-grade or afternoon fever, malar flush, warm palms and soles, dry mouth and red lips, dark red and dry tongue with little coating, constipation, scanty and dark urine, and small rapid pulse are relatively predominant.

The following formula is prescribed to tonify the Yin and dissolve the dampness and remove blood stasis.

Shi Wu Tang Jia Jian.

Constituents:

Milk veteh    60g
Chinese angelica    30g
Unpeeled root of herbaceous peony    30g
Chuanxiong    30g
Root of Zhejiang figwort    30g
Fresh or dried root of rehmannia    30g

Asian puccoon   30g
Broom cypress fruit   60g
Cicada slough   30g
Skullcap   12g
Common duckweed 15g
Jingjie   12g
Shechuangzi   12g
Sophora flavescens   15g

Decoction and dosage is the same.

*2. Acupuncture therapy*

Main points: LI11 Quchi, Sp10 Xuehai, G20 Fengchi and Sp6 Sanyinjiao.
Auxiliary points: GV14 Dazhui, S36 Zusanli and LI4 Hegu.
Method: All the above points can be punctured before or during the attack. Each time two or three of each of the main and auxiliary points are punctured with strong stimulation. The needles are retained for 30 minutes and the therapy is given once daily.

*3. Ear-acupuncture therapy*

Points: Urticaria Zone Pt, Lung Pt, Adrenal Gland Pt, Endocrine Pt and Shenmen Pt.
Method: Each time three or four of the above points are punctured with strong stimulation. The needles are retained for 2 to 4 hours and the therapy is given once daily.

*4. Point injection therapy*

Points: B13 Feishu, Sp10 Xuehai, LI11 Quchi and S36 Zusanli.
Drugs: 5% Chinese angelica solution and Vitamin B1.
Method: Either of the above drugs can be prescribed and each of the above points is injected with 0.3 to 0.5 millilitre of the solution. The therapy is given once daily.

# 2. FURUNCULOSIS (BOILS) AND CARBUNCLES

## GENERAL CONSIDERATION

A furuncle (boil) is a deep-seated infection (abscess) involving the entire hair follicle and adjacent subcutaneous tissue. The most common sites of occurrence are the hairy parts exposed to irritation and friction, pressure, moisture or to the plugging action of petroleum products. Because the lesions are autoinoculable, they are often multiple. Thorough investigation usually fails to uncover a predisposing cause, although an occasional patient may have uncontrolled diabetes mellitus, nephritis, or other debilitating disease. Groups may be subject to epidemics.

A carbuncle is several furuncles developing in adjoining hair follicles and coalescing to form a conglomerate, deeply situated mass with multiple drainage points.

In traditional Chinese medicine, the concept and understanding of the condition is the same as that in Western medicine.

## CLINICAL MANIFESTATIONS

The extreme tenderness and pain are due to pressure on nerve endings, particularly in areas where there is little room for swelling of underlying structures. The pain, fever and malaise are more severe with carbuncles than with furuncles. The follicular abscess is either rounded or conical. It gradually enlarges, becomes fluctuant and then softens and opens spontaneously after a few days to 1 or 2 weeks to discharge a core of necrotic tissue and pus. The inflammation occasionally subsides before necrosis occurs.

There also may be slight leukocytosis.

## DIAGNOSIS

Essentials of diagnosis.

• Extremely painful inflammatory swelling of a hair follicle that forms an abscess.

    • Primary predisposing debiliting disease sometimes present.

    • Coagulase-positive staphylococcus aureus is the causative organism.

## TREATMENT

### I. Treatment in Western medicine.

*1. Specific measures*

Systemic anti-infection agents are indicated (chosen on the basis of cultures and sensitivity tests if possible). Sodium cloxacillin or erythromycin, 1g daily by mouth for 10 days, is usually effective. Cephalexin is an effective alternative drug. Minocycline may be effective against strains of staphyloccoci resistant to other antibiotics.

Strains of pathogenic staphylococci may carry a plasmid or episome, causing resistance to antibiotics such as erythromycin.

*2. Local measures*

Immobilize the part and avoid overmanipulation of inflamed areas. Use moist heat to help larger lesions "localize." Use surgical incision and debridement after the lesions are "mature." Do not incise deeply. Apply anti-infective ointment and bandage the area loosely during drainage. It is not necessary to incise and drain an acute staphylococcal paronychia. Inserting a flat metal spatula or sharpened hardwood stick into the nail fold where it adjoins the nail will release pus from a mature lesion.

### II. Treatment in traditional Chinese medicine.

*1. Herb therapy*

Furuncle is an acute suppurative follicle lesion of the skin, usually starting in a hair follicle or a sebaceous gland and its surrounding tissue. It is one of the commonest inflammatory lesions of the skin, characterized by its superficial situation in any location of the body, localized redness, swelling and pain. The treatment in traditional Chinese medicine is intended to dissipate heat and detoxify the body with Wu Wei Xiao Du Yin Jia Jian.

The constituents are:

Honeysuckle flower   60g
Weeping forsythia (fruit)   60g
Skullcap   12g
Chonglou   20g
Unpeeled root of herbaceous peony   30g
Root of Zhejiang figwort   30g
Chinese goldthread   10g
Skunk bugbane   12g
Dandelion   30g
Chinese violet   30g
Giant knotweed   30g
Chinese angelica   30g
Chinese honeylocuist spine   12g
Wild chrysanthemum   15g

Decoction and dosage. All the above herbs are put together into a boiler to be simmered twice and then the broth of each mixed, half of the mixed broth each time, twice a day. Two to four doses are prescribed.

*2. Acupuncture therapy*

Application of the fresh leaves of rumex madaio makino on the inflamed areas is also very effective. The leaves are collected and smashed into paste for application one or twice a day for some days.

# Chapter XI
# DISEASES OF THE EYE, EAR, NOSE AND THROAT

## 1. CONJUNCTIVITIS

### GENERAL CONSIDERATION

Conjunctivitis is one of the most common eye diseases which may be acute or chronic. Most cases are exogenous and due to bacterial, viral or chlamydial infection though endogenous inflammation may occur. Other causes are allergy, chemical irritations and fungal or parasitic infection. The mode of transmission of infectious conjunctivitis is usually the direct contact via fingers, towels, handkerchiefs to the fellow eye or to other persons.

Bacterial Conjunctivitis. The organisms found most commonly in bacterial conjunctivitis are streptococcus pneumonia, staphylococcus aureus, Koch-weeks bacillus and Morax-Axenfeld bacillus.

Viral Conjunctivitis. One of the commonest causes of viral conjunctivitis is adenovirus type 3, which is usually associated with pharyngitis, fever, malaise and preauricular adenopathy.

In traditional Chinese medicine, this condition is termed "Feng Huo Yan Tong," "Feng Re Yan" or "Huo Yan," which is thought to be caused by pathogenic wind and heat. It may become epidemic.

### CLINICAL MANIFESTATIONS

Bacterial Conjunctivitis. There is no pain or blurring of vision. The disease is usually self-limited, lasting about 10 to 14 days if untreated.

Viral Conjunctivitis. Locally, the palpebral conjunctiva is red and there is a copious watery discharge and scanty exudate. Children are more often affected than adults and contaminated swimming pools are sometimes the source of infection.

### DIAGNOSIS

According to the symptoms and signs, bacterial conjunctivitis produces a copious purulent discharge. There is no pain or blurring of vision. In viral conjunctivitis, the palpebral conjunctiva is red and there is a copious watery discharge and scanty exudate.

## TREATMENT

### I. Management in Western medicine.

For bacterial conjunctivitis.

A sulfonamide or antibiotic ointment, instilled locally 3 times daily, will usually clear the infection in 2 to 3 days. Antibiotic-corticosteroid combinations are not advisable.

For viral conjunctivitis.

There is no specific treatment for viral conjunctivitis, although local sulfonamide therapy may prevent secondary bacterial infection. The disease usually lasts at least 2 weeks.

### II. Management in traditional Chinese medicine.

*1. Herb therapy*

According to the theory of traditional Chinese medicine, the eyes are thought to be the windows of the liver. Certain physiologic and pathologic changes of the liver may manifest as disorders of the eyes.

As the palpebral conjunctiva is red with copious watery discharge, scanty exudate, sudden onset, rapid pulse and yellowish coating of the tongue, it is thought to be caused by the hepatic fire. The general rule for treatment is to purge the liver fire, and the effective herb formula is Lun Dan Run Gan Tang Jia Jian.

Constituents:

Rough gentian (root)  20g
Capejasmine  12g
Skullcap  12g
Chinese thorowax  15g
Oriental water plantain  12g
Asiatic plantain seed  25g
Chinese angelica  20g
Fresh or dried root of rehmannia  20g
Chrysanthemun  15g
Dandelion  25g
Chinese violet  30g
Honeysuckle flower  25g
Forsythia suspensa  25g

Decoction and dosage. All the above herbs are put together to be simmered twice and then the broth of each mixed. Half of the mixed broth each time, twice a day. Six doses are prescribed.

*2. Acupuncture therapy*

Main points: B1 Jingming and Taiyang (extra).

Auxiliary points: G20 Fengchi, TE23 Sizukong, B2 Zanzhu, S1 Chengqi and LI4 Hegu.

Method: For acute conjunctivitis, first puncture B2 Zanzhu and TE23 Sizukong, then Taiyang (extra), and finally G20 Fengchi, B1 Jingming and LI4 Hegu. Taiyang (extra) is punctured to cause bleeding so as to relieve the congestion of the bulbar conjunctiva. For chronic conjuctivitis, first puncture all the main points and then one or two of the auxiliary points. The therapy is given once daily.

*3. Ear-acupuncture therapy*

Points: Liver Pt, Eye Pt, Eye Pt 1 and Eye Pt 2.

Method: All the above points are punctured with moderate stimulation. The needles are retained for 30 minutes and the therapy is given once daily.

## 2. EPISTAXIS

### GENERAL CONSIDERATION

The most common sites of nasal bleeding are the mucosal vessels over the cartilaginous nasal septum and the anterior tip of the inferior turbinate. Bleeding is usually due to external trauma, nose picking, nasal infection, or drying of the nasal mucosa. Over 5% of nosebleeds originate posteriorly in the nose, where the bleeding site cannot be seen; these can cause great problems in management. If the blood drains into the pharynx and is swallowed, nosebleed may escape diagnosis. In these cases, bloody vomitus may be the first clue.

Underlying causes of nosebleed such as blood dyscrasias, hypertension, hemorrhagic disease, nasal tumors, and certain infectious diseases (measles or rheumatic fever) must be considered in any case of recurrent or profuse nosebleed without obvious causes.

In traditional Chinese medicine, the condition is termed "Bi Niu," which simply means epistaxis, and is thought to be caused by dry lungs.

### CLINICAL MANIFESTATIONS

Bleeding of the nasal cavity. It chiefly occurs in infants and is manifested as redness, itchiness, pain and ulceration of the nares, or drying of the nasal mucosa.

### DIAGNOSIS

• Must rule out blood dyscrasias, hypertension, hemorrhagic disease, nasal tumor and certain infectious diseases.

• The Patient should be adequately examined for any contributing systemic disease.

### TREATMENT

**I. Management in Western medicine.**

Local measures:

A. For anterior epistaxis, pressure over the area for 5 minutes is often sufficient to stop bleeding. This may be combined with packing the bleeding nostril with 0.25% phenylephrine or 1:1000 epinephrine solution.

After active bleeding has stopped, a cotton pledget moistened with a topical anesthetic applied to the bleeding area will provide anesthesia for cauterization with a chronic acid bead, trichloroacetic acid, or an eletrocautery. After cauterization, lubrication with petrolatum helps prevent crusting. A second cauterization is infrequently necessary.

If the source of bleeding is not accessible to cauterization or is not controlled by cauterization, the nasal cavity must be packed. After maximum shrinkage of the mucosa has been achieved with a suitable decongestant and typical anesthesia, the nasal cavity can be tightly packed with help—an inch gauze lubricated with petrolatum or cod liver oil. Pack the gauze into the nose in layers, starting either in the vault or on the floor of the nasal cavity. The packing may be left in place as long as 5 to 6 days if necessary. The patient should be given analgesics for pain and antibiotic medications for suppurative otitis media and sinusitis as needed.

B. For posterior epistaxis, posterior bleeding can sometimes be controlled only by means of a posterior nasal pack. This accomplishes 2 things: it compresses and controls bleeding sites in the nasopharynx or posterior choana, and it prevents very firm anterior packing from being dislodged into the pharynx.

## II. Management in traditional Chinese medicine.

In traditional Chinese medicine, the nose is understood as the opening of the lungs. Hence, the nosebleed is usually thought to be caused by the pulmonic heat. The general rule of treatment is to dissipate the heat and to cool blood.

*1. Herb therapy*
A. Xi Jiao Di Huang Tang Jia Jian.
Constituents:

Buffalo horn   30g
Fresh or dried root of rehmannia   30g
Unpeeled root of herbaceous peony   30g
Root-bark of peony   15g
Skullcap   12g
Cogongrass rhizome   50g
Field thistle   25g
Node of lotus rhizome   25g
Capejasmine   12g
Donkey-hide gelation   15g
Root of pseudo-ginseng   2g

Decoction and dosage. All the above herbs are put together into a boiler to be simmered twice and then the broth of each mixed, half of the mixed broth each time, twice a day. Two to four doses are prescribed.

B. 30 grams of Chinese parasol seeds is ground into fine powder and taken with water three times daily. We tried this in 320 cases and found it was very effective in 240. In other 80 cases, though the effect was not remarkable, it certainly relieved the condition to some degree.

*2. Acupuncture therapy*

Points: LI20 Yingxiang, L11 Shaoshang, GV23 Shangxing and LI4 Hegu.
Method: All the above points are punctured with moderate stimulation and the needles are retained for 20 minutes.

## 3. SIMPLE PHARYNGITIS

### GENERAL CONSIDERATION

Acute simple (catarrhal) pharyngitis is an acute inflammation of the mucosa of the pharynx that to some extent involves the lymphatic structures. It usually occurs as part of an upper respiratory tract disorder that may also affect the nose, sinuses, larynx and trachea. The most common causes are bacterial or viral infection and rarely, it is due to inhalation of irritant gases or ingestion of irritant liquids. Pharyngitis may occur as part of the syndrome of an acute specific infection.

The inflammation may be diffuse or localized. Drying of the mucosa occurs in pharyngitis sicca.

In traditional Chinese medicine, the disorder is called "Feng Ren Hou Bi," which means sore throat due to pathogenic wind and heat.

### CLINICAL MANIFESTATIONS

In acute pharyngitis, the throat is dry and sore. Systemic symptoms are fever and malaise. The pharyngeal mucosa is red and slightly swollen, with thick and sticky mucus. The disease lasts only a few days.

Chronic pharyngitis may produce few symptoms, such as throat dryness with thick mucus and cough; or recurrent acute episodes of more severe throat pain, dull hyperemia and mild swelling of the mucosa and thick tenacious mucus, often in the hypopharynx.

### DIAGNOSIS

- The throat is dry and sore.
- Some patients with fever and malaise.
- The pharyngeal mucosa is red and slightly swollen with thick or sticky mucus.

### TREATMENT

**I. Treatment in Western medicine**

The treatment of acute pharyngitis in western medicine is symptomatic; rest, light diet, analgesics, and warm, nonirritating gargles or throat irrigations. Antibiotics may be used for initial or complicating bacterial infection.

Chronic pharyngitis is treated by removing underlying causes such as infections of the nose, sinuses, or tonsils and by restricting irritants such as alcohol, spicy foods and tobacco. Local removal of the tenacious secretion with suction or saline irrigation and application of 2% silver nitrate are helpful.

**II. Management in traditional Chinese medicine**

Because sore throat is due to wind and heat, the patient often complains of fever, mild chilly sensation, slight thirst, and the pharyngeal mucosa is red and slightly swollen with redness of the edges and tip of the tongue with thin yellowish coating, superficial and rapid pulse, etc.

The general rule of treatment is to relieve the condition with the cold pungent herbs. The effective formula is Yin Xiao San Jia Jian.

Constituents:

Honeysuckle flower   30g
Forsythia suspensa  30g
Achene of great burdock   12g
Chrysanthemum   12g
Root of Zhejiang figwort   20g
Fresh or dried root of rehmannia   30g
Tuber of dwarf lilyturf   30g
Skullcap   12g
Root of balloonflower   12g
Puff-ball   12g
Chinese thorowax   15g
Peppermint   10g

Decoction and dosage is the same.

In addition, the ready made herb pills such as Lu Shen Pills and Nu Huang Xian Yan Pills are all very effective for chronic pharyngitis.

# Chapter XII
# STOMATOLOGICAL DISEASES

## 1. APHTHOUS ULCER

### GENERAL CONSIDERATION

An aphthous ulcer is a shallow mucosal ulcer with flat, fairly even borders surrounded by erythema. The ulcer is often covered with a pseudomembrane. It has never been adequately demonstrated that this lesion is due to a virus or any other specific chemical, physical or microbial agent. One or more ulcers may be present, and they tend to be recurrent.

It is called oral ulcer in traditional Chinese medicine, and is usually caused by upward steaming of the stomach heat.

### CLINICAL MANIFESTATIONS

They are often painful; nuts, chocolates, and irritants such as citrus fruits often cause flare-ups of aphthous ulceration, but abstinence will not prevent recurrence. Stresses of various types have also been shown to be contributory. Aphthous ulcer may be associated with inflammatory bowel disease, Behcet's syndrome, infectious mononucleosis and prolonged fever. The diagnosis depends mainly upon ruling out similar but more readily identifiable disease, a history of recurrence, and inspection of the ulcer.

### DIAGNOSIS

- The aphthous ulcer is usually recurrent.
- Inspection of the ulcer. The ulcer is a shallow mucosal ulcer with flat, fairly even borders surrounded by erythema.
- The diagnosis depends mainly upon ruling out similar but more readily identifiable disease.

### TREATMENT

**I. Management in Western medicine.**

Bland mouth rinses and hydrocortisone—antibiotic ointment reduce pain and encourage healing. Hydrocortisone in an adhesive base (orabase) has been particularly useful. Sedatives, analgesics and vitamins may help indirectly. Vaccines and gamma globulins have not proved significantly beneficial. Although caustics relieve pain by cauterizing the fine nerve endings, they also cause necrosis and scar tissue. Systemic antibiotics are contraindicated. Systemic corticosteroids in high doses for a short period of time may be very helpful for severe debilitating recurrent attacks.

Healing, which usually occurs in 1 to 3 weeks, may be only slightly accelerated by treatment. Occasionally, aphthous ulcers take the form of periadenitis, in which they are larger, persist sometimes for months, and may leave a scar. This form can be confused with carcinoma.

## II. Management in traditional Chinese medicine.

Oral ulcer is thought to be caused by excessive heat in the stomach, with the manifestations such as polydipsia, preference for cold drinks, fetid breath, ulceration of the mouth, swelling and pain of the gums, burning sensation of the epigastrium, scanty dark urine, constipation, red tongue with thick yellowish coating. The principle of the treatment is to dissipate heat and detoxify the body, and the most effective formula often prescribed is Qing Wei San Jia Jian.

Constituents:

Skunk bugbane   12g
Chinese goldthread   10g
Chinese angelica   15g
Fresh and dried root of rehmannia   30g
Root-bark of peony   15g
Gypsum   30g
Dyers woad root 30g
Dyers woad leaf   30g
Honeysuckle flower   30g
Root-bark of peony   15g
Root of Zhejiang figwort   30g
Skullcap   12g

Decoction and dosage. All the above herbs are put together into a boiler to be simmered twice and then the broth of each mixed, half of the mixed broth each time, twice a day. Two to four doses are prescribed.

# Chapter XIII
# DISEASES OF THE NERVOUS SYSTEM

## 1. PERIPHERAL FACIAL PARALYSIS
### (Bell's palsy)

### GENERAL CONSIDERATION

Bell's palsy is a paralysis of the muscles of one side of the face, sometimes precipitated by exposure to chill or trauma. It may occur at any age but is slightly more common in the age group from 20 to 50.

In traditional Chinese medicine, the onset of the illness is thought to be due to derangement of Qi and blood and malnutrition of the channels caused by invasion of the channels and collaterals in the facial region by pathogenic wind-cold or phlegm.

### CLINICAL MANIFESTATIONS

On the affected side are incomplete closing of the eye, lacrimation, drooping of the angle of the mouth, salivation and inability to frown, raise the eyebrow, close the eye, blow out the cheek, show the teeth or whistle. There may be pain in the mastoid region or headache.

### DIAGNOSIS

The diagnosis is based on the symptoms, but must rule out cerebrovascular accidents (strokes) and intracranial tumors. The peripheral facial paralysis patients are specially unable to frown and raise the eyebrow, close the eye of the paralyzed side. The intracranial tumors can be ruled out by X-ray examination.

### TREATMENT

**I. Treatment in Western medicine.**

Keep the face warm and avoid further exposure, especially to wind and dust. Protect the eye with a patch if necessary. Support the face with a tape or wire anchored at the angle of the mouth and looped about the ear. Electric stimulation (every other day after the 14th day) may be used to help prevent muscle atrophy. Gentle upward massage of the involved muscles for 5 to 10 minutes 2 to 3 times daily may help to maintain muscle tone. Heat from an infrared lamp may hasten recovery.

Prednisone therapy has been reported to be effective but is of doubtful value.

## II. Treatment in traditional Chinese medicine.

### 1. Acupuncture therapy

Points: TE17 Yifeng, S4 Dicang, S6 Jiache, G14 Yangbai, Taiyang (extra), LI4 Hegu, SI18 Guanliao and S7 Xiaguan.

Method: 3 to 5 of the above points are selected for each treatment and the therapy is given once daily. S4 Dicang and S6 Jiache are punctured together with one needle inserted horizontally from S4 Dicang to S6 Jiache. The following points can also be added to the formula according to the symptoms: G20 Fengchi for headache; S40 Fenglong for profuse sputum; B2 Zanzhu and TE23 Sizhukong for difficulty in frowning and raising the eyebrow; B2 Zanzhu, B1 Jingming, B15 Tongziliao, Yuyao (extra) and TE23 Sizhukong for incomplete closing of the eye lids; LI20 Yingxiang for difficulty in sniffling; GV26 Renzhong for deviation of the philtrum; S3 Juliao for inability to show the teeth; G2 Tinghui for tinnitus and deafness; SI4 Wangu for tenderness at the mastoid region; and Liv3 Taichong for twitching of the eyelid and the mouth.

### 2. Herb therapy

Zhi Jing San Jia Jian.

Constituents:

Scorpion  2.5g
Fangfeng  13g
Larvia of silkworm of rehmannia    10g
Baifuzi  10g
Milk veteh   30g
Chinese angelica    15g
Unpeeled root of herbaceous peony    15g
Chuanxiong   15g
Peach kernel    12g
Safflower  12g

Decoction and dosage. All the above herbs make a dose and six to ten doses are prescribed with one dose daily. Each dose is simmered twice and then the broth of each mixed, half of the mixed broth each time, twice a day.

### 3. Electro-acupuncture therapy

Main points: Qianzheng (extra) and CV17 Yifeng.

Auxiliary points: G14 Yangbai, Taiyang (extra) and S4 Dicang.

Method: One of the main points and two or three of the auxiliary points are prescribed each time. The main point is connected to the negative pole of the electro-acupuncture machine, and the auxiliary points to the positive pole. The frequency is adjusted to 20 to 30 times per minute with an output which can just cause the muscular twitch on the affected side. The treatment lasts for 15 minutes and is repeated once every other day. Ten times makes a course.

The patient can be assured that recovery usually occurs in 2 to 8 weeks (or up to 1 to 2 years in older patients). In the vast majority of cases, partial or complete recovery occurs. When recovery is partial, contractures may develop on the paralyzed side. Recurrence on the same or the opposite side is occasionally reported. Acupuncture therapy is very effective for this condition.

## 2. VIRAL ENCEPHALITIS

### GENERAL CONSIDERATION

Encephalitis may be defined as an inflammatory process of the CNS that results in altered function of various portions of the brain and spinal cord and is usually accompanied by signs of systemic infection.

Viral encephalitis may be characterized by: 1. A mild abortive infection; 2. A type of illness clinically indistinguishable from aseptic meningitis; and 3. A severe involvement of the CNS. The latter is often characterized by a sudden onset, high fever, meningeal signs, stupor, disorientation, tremors, convulsions, spasticity, coma and death. Case fatality ranges from 1% to 34.9%. The sequelae are more common in infants. A specific diagnosis can be made either by demonstrating a rise in the level of antibody in the serum of the convalescent patient or by isolating a virus from the CNS or CSF.

In traditional Chinese medicine, the condition is considered to be caused by epidemic Qi, a pathogenic factor of high infectivity. The terms of diagnosis are "acute or fulminating infectious disease in summer," or "summer-heat convulsion," or "acute febrile disease with prolonged onset."

### CLINICAL MANIFESTATIONS

There are many types of viral encephalitides. They vary from benign forms, resembling aseptic meningitis, lasting a few days and are followed by complete recovery to fulminating encephalitis with the clinical manifestations of paresis, sensory changes, convulsions, increased intracranial pressure, coma and death.

The onset of viral encephalitis may be sudden or gradual and is marked by fever, headache, dizziness, vomiting, apathy and stiffness of the neck. Ataxia, tremors, mental confusion, speech difficulties, stupor or hyperexcitability, delirium, convulsions and coma, and death may follow. In some cases there may be a prodromal period of 1 to 4 days characterized by chills and fever, headache, malaise, sore throat, conjunctivitis, and pains in the extremities and abdomen followed by encephalitic signs just mentioned. Abortive forms with headache and fever only or a syndrome resembling aseptic meningitis may occur.

The many variations in the clinical patterns of encephalitis depend on the distribution, location and concentration of neuronal lesions. Ocular palsies and ptosis are uncommon. Cerebellar incoordination is seen. Flaccid paralysis of the extremities resembling that of poliomyelitis is sometimes encountered. Paralysis of the shoulder girdle muscle is described as a singular feature of a tick-bone encephalitis.

The CSF is clear and manometric readings of pressure vary from normal to markedly elevated. As a rule, pleocytosis of 40 to 400 cells, chiefly mononuclear, is found. The protein and glucose values may be slightly elevated or normal.

## DIAGNOSIS

A diagnosis of acute encephalitis is indicated by the clinical findings. The circumstances in which the disease occurs are important. The specific type of encephalitis can be determined only by isolation and identification of the virus or by demonstration of the formation of or rise of level of antibody in convalescence. Arboviruses are rarely detected in the CSF, blood or other materials during life. It is generally fruitless and inappropriate to search for them except in CNS tissue removed with sterile precautions at necropsy. A serologic diagnosis may be reached by means of the complement fixation or hemagglutination-inhibition test. Paired serum specimens are necessary. The first should be drawn as soon after onset as possible and the second, 2 or 3 weeks later.

## TREATMENT

### I. Treatment in Western medicine.

Although there has been little to offer in the way of specific treatment for viral encephalitis in the past, recent evidence indicates that antiviral chemotherapy may be worth using in patients with encephalitis caused by herpes simplex virus. It appears that a number of compounds interfere with DNA metabolism and inhibit multiplication of herpes simplex virus. Herpes simplex virus encephalitis carries a high fatality rate of 35%, which may justify the use of potentially toxic drugs. Clinical manifestations of temporal lobe involvement are common and may be supported by electroencephalograms and brain scan. It is recommended that the diagnosis be established by biopsy of the involved temporal lobe for isolation of herpes simplex virus or by identification of herpes virus antigen with fluorescent-antibody methods before treatment is begun. Treatment is most beneficial when given early in the course of the disease before brain damage occurs from infection or increased intracranial pressure.

The use of antimicrobial agents to prevent infection is contraindicated because it predisposes to infection by resistant organisms. The use of tetracycline should be avoided especially because it can give rise to intracranial hypertension.

There is no evidence that steroids are beneficial in the treatment of viral encephalitis. Systemic and intracranial hypertension and other well-known side effects should discourage the use of steroids in viral encephalitis.

The use of mannitol and other hypertonic solutions may effect a temporary drop in intracranial pressure, but the usual rebound effect diminishes their value.

Immune serum globulin, whole blood and pooled plasma are of no value in the treatment of encephalitis. There is no evidence that vaccinia immune globulin alters the course of postvaccinal encephalitis.

The usual sedatives are indicated for hyperexcitability and convulsion. Hyperthermia is usually controlled by giving the patient tepid sponge baths or by using an ice blanket. Intravenous infusions may be necessary to maintain proper balance of water and electrolytes. Severe involvement of the medulla, with impairment of swallowing and accumulation of secretions in the throat and paralysis of the vocal cords or respiratory muscles, should be treated in the same way as that of bulbar poliomyelitis. If gentle aspiration fails to keep the airway open, tracheostomy is indicated. Respiratory support may be necessary for patients with respiratory paralysis, either peripheral or central in origin.

## II. Treatment in traditional Chinese medicine.

### 1. Herb therapy

A. For acute febrile disease with prolonged onset.

Acute febrile diseases with rather prolonged latencies after the pathogenic warm factor entering the body any time in the four seasons is characterized by the symptom complex of internal heat at the onset. The chief symptoms are fever, headache, perspiration, chilly sensation, pain of the throat, thirst, stiffness of the neck, mental confusion, delirium, convulsions. thin white or slight yellowish coating of the tongue and rapid pulse. The principle for treatment is to purify the Qi with pungent-cold drugs and to detoxify the body. The formula of first choice is Bai Hu Tang Jia Jian.

Constituents:

Gypsum  60g
Root of Zhejiang figwort  30g
Tuber of dwarf lilyturf  30g
Fresh or dried rehmannia  30g
Rhizome of wind-weed  12g
Honeysuckle flower 30g
Weeping forsythia (fruit)  30g
Common red rhizome  30g
Dryers woad root   30g
Dryers woad leaf   30g
Cicada slough   20g
Larva of a silkworm wirh batrytis   10g
Licorice root   6g

Decoction and dosage. All the above herbs make a dose and six to ten doses are prescribed with one dose daily. Each dose is simmered twice and then the broth of each mixed, half of the mixed broth each time, twice a day.

B. For acute febrile disease with the invasion of the heat into the pericardium. The onset of this type is either sudden or gradual and marked by fever, headache, mental confusion, stupor, delirium, tremors, yellow coating of the tongue with dark red colour, and full pulse. The treatment is to purge the pathogenic fire and calm the wind with Qing Ying Tang Jia Jian.

Constituents:

Gypsum  60g
Rhizome of wind-weed  12g
Fresh or dried rehmannia  20g

Root of Zhejiang figwort 30g
Root-bark of peony 15g
Dyers woad root 30g
Dyers woad leaf 30g
Rhubarb 10g
Jack-in-the-pulpit 12g
Tabasheer 12g
Earthworm 15g
Scorpion 15 pieces
Centipede 1 or 2 pieces
Buffalo horn 30g

Decoction and dosage is the same.

C. For acute febrile disease due to the disturbance of the heart by phlegmatic fire. Thermal pathogen in combination with "phlegm" causes mental disturbances. The main symptoms are mental confusion, delirium, mania and excitability, or spitting sputum and saliva, red tongue with yellowish and glossy coating, slippery and rapid pulse. The treatment is to reduce phlegm for resuscitation with Dao Tan Tang Jia Jian.

Constituents:

Dried old orange peel 12g
Pinellia 12g
Tuckahoe 10g
Licorice root 6g
Jack-in-the-pulpit 12g
Fruit of immature citron or trifoliate orange 12g
Tabasheer 12g
Grass-leaved sweetflag 12g
Root-tuber of aromatic turmeric 12g
Bamboo shavings 12g
Musk 0.06g
Bamboo juice 3 or 4 spoonful

Decoction and dosage is the same.

D. For acute febrile diseases caused by the inward invasion of the weak wind. Diseases due to the impairment of Yin and deficiency of blood manifest poor maintenance of muscles and tendons, and produce symptoms simulating the wind movements such as dizziness, convulsions or tremor, flushed face, hot palms and soles, dysphoria, restlessness, insomnia, dry throat and mouth, dark red tongue with reduced saliva, weak and rapid pulse. The treatment is to calm the "wind" through nourishing the Yin. The commonly used formula is Da Ding Feng Zu Tang Jia Jian.

Constituents:

Root of herbaceous 30g
Donkey-hide gelatin 12g
Tortoise plastron 20g
Dried rehmannia 20g

Fructus cannabis  20g
Fruit of Chinese magnaliavine  20g
Tuber of dwarf lilyturf  30g
Oyster  30g
Turtle-shell 30g
Radix glycyrrhizae  6g
Egg core  6g

Decoction and dosage is the same.

Certain ready-made herb pills such as An Gong Niu Huang Pill, Niu Huang Qing Xin Pill, Zi Xue Dan and Zhi Biao Dan are also very effective for the conditions.

*2. Acupuncture therapy*

A. For paralysis of the upper limbs.

Points: LI15 Jianyu, LI11 Quchi, LI4 Hegu and TE5 Waiguan.

B. For paralysis of the lower limbs.

Points: S31 Biguan, S36 Zusanli, S41 Jiexi, G30 Huantiao, G34 Yanglingquan and G39 Xuanzhong.

C. For convulsion.

Points: CV12 Zhongwan, CV4 Guanyuan, S36 Zusanli, Liv13 Zhangmen and Yintang (extra).

D. For eye deviation.

Points: LI4 Hegu, B1 Jingming, G20 Fengchi, Taiyang (extra) and Liv2 Xingjian.

Method: All the points are punctured with moderate stimulation and the needles are retained for 20 minutes. The therapy is given once daily.


# 3. CEREBROVASCULAR ACCIDENTS

## GENERAL CONSIDERATION

Cerebrovascular accident, or stroke, is a focal neurologic disorder due to a pathologic process in a blood vessel. In most cases the onset is abrupt and evolution rapid, and symptoms reach a peak within seconds, minutes or hours. Partial or complete recovery may occur over a period of hours to months.

Occlusion of a cerebral artery by thrombosis or embolism results in a cerebral infarction with its associated clinical effects. Other conditions may on occasion also produce cerebral infarction and thus may be confused with cerebral thrombosis or embolism. These include cerebral venous thrombosis, cerebral arteritis, systemic hypotension, reactions to cerebral angiography, and transient cerebral ischemia.

Cerebral hemorrhage is usually caused by rupture of an arteriosclerotic cerebral vessel. Subarachnoid hemorrhage is usually due to rupture of a congenitally weak blood vessel or aneurysm.

Transient cerebral ischemia may also occur without producing a cerebral infarction. Premonitory recurrent focal cerebral ischemic attacks may occur and are apt to be in a repetitive pattern in a given case. Attacks may last for 10 seconds to 1 hour, but the average duration is 2 to 10 minutes. As many as several hundred such attacks may occur. In some instances of transient ischemia, the neurologic deficit may last up to 20 hours.

Narrowing of the extracranial arteries (particularly the internal carotid artery at its origin in the neck and, in some cases, the intrathoracic arteries) by arteriosclerotic patches has been incriminated in a significant number of cases of transient cerebral ischemias and infarction.

In traditional Chinese medicine, the disease is considered to be caused by stirring wind arising from hyperactivity of Yang in the liver which results from exasperation or agitation accompanied with disturbance of the Zang-fu organs, Qi and blood imbalance of Yin and Yang and dysfunction of the channels and collaterals. Another factor is endogenous wind caused by phlegm-heat after over-indulgence in alcohol and fatty diet.

## CLINICAL MANIFESTATIONS

Early phase. Variable degrees and types occur. The onset may be violent, with the patient falling to the ground and lying inert like a person in deep sleep, with flushed face, stertorous or cheyne-stroke respirations, full and slow pulse, and one arm and leg usually flaccid. Death may occur in a few hours or days. Lesser grades of stroke may consist of slight derangement of speech, thought, motion, sensation, or vision. Consciousness need not be altered. Symptoms may last seconds to minutes or longer or may persist unremittingly for an indefinite period. Some degree of recovery is usual.

Premonitory symptoms may include headache, dizziness, drowsiness, and mental confusion. Focal premonitory symptoms are more likely to occur with thrombosis.

Generalized neurologic signs are most common with cerebral hemorrhage and include fever, headache, vomiting, convulsion, and coma. Nuchal rigidity is frequent with subarachnoid hemorrhage or intracerebral hemorrhage. Mental changes are commonly noted in the period following a stroke and may include confusion, disorientation and memory defects.

## DIAGNOSIS

Essentials of diagnosis.
• Sudden onset of neurologic complaints varying from focal motor or hypesthesia and speech defects to profound coma.
• May be associated with vomiting, convulsions or headaches.
• Nuchal rigidity frequently found.

## TREATMENT

### I. Treatment in Western medicine.

1. *Acute stage or onset*
A. General measures.
The patient should be placed at complete bed rest and handled carefully to avoid injury. Give tranquilizers or sedatives as necessary to control agitation.

B. Anticoagulant therapy.

Maintenance on anticoagulant therapy has been advocated for treatment and prevention of cerebral thrombosis or insufficiency of the carotid or vertebral-basilar system. The evidence is more promising for transient cerebral ischemia. The risk of hemorrhage, particularly in hypertensive patients, is great.

C. Antiplatelet agents.

Several studies have shown that aspirin may reduce the risk of transient ischemic attack and stroke, particularly in men. Aspirin 0.3/per day.

D. Surgery. Narrowing of the extracranial arteries as shown on angiography may be an indication for surgical correction.

*2. Special problems in hemiplegic patients*

A. Care of the paralyzed upper extremity.

In most cases no useful function returns to the paralyzed upper extremity. With the uninvolved hand, the patient should move the paralyzed fingers, wrist, and elbow through the full range of motion twice a day. Treatment of painful shoulder consists of analgesics, immobilization, and gentle range of motion exercises.

B. Treatment of aphasia.

If aphasia occurs, speech therapy should be started as soon as possible. If secondary or receptive aphasia is present, the above program may be rendered extremely difficult, since it is based on the ability of the patient to understand direction.

C. Care of hemianopia.

If hemianopia is present, the patient should be trained to turn the head to the hemianopic side in order to bring the visual field within view.

D. Care of sphincters.

Some hemiplegics are incontinent in the early phase. The patient should be reminded to empty the bladder voluntarily at hourly intervals. These intervals can be gradually increased.

E. Organic brain syndrome.

Impaired mentation is an obstacle to the rehabilitation program. The confusion may be present at one time and absent at another, and advantage should be taken of the patient's lucid period. Organic brain syndrome occurs more often in patients who had several strokes. The patient's mental state improves considerably during an active rehabilitation program.

F. Medications.

All central nervous system depressant drugs, even in small doses, may have a detrimental effect on the stroke patient. They may cause or aggravate confusion, aphasia, lack of balance and incontinence. If used as hypotensive or anticonvulsive agents, they should be replaced if possible by nondepressant drugs. On the other hand, central nervous system stimulant drugs can help improve function in the confused and depressed patient.

## II. Treatment in traditional Chinese medicine.

*2. Acupuncture therapy*

Acupuncture therapy is indispensable at the stage of recovery and convalescence.

There are two types of windstroke according to the degree of severity: the severe type and the mild type.

The severe type. In this type, the Zang-fu organs are attacked and the symptoms are manifested in the channels, collaterals and the viscerae. The severe type can further be divided into two subtypes:

A. The tense syndrome. The chief manifestations of this type are sudden collapse, coma, staring eyes, clenched fists and jaws, redness of face and ears, gurgling with sputum, coarse breathing, retention of urine, and constipation, wiry and rolling forceful pulse. The prescription for puncture is:

Main points: GV26 Renzhong, GV20 Baihui and K1 Yongquan.

Auxiliary points: S6 Jiache, S7 Xiaguan and LI4 Hegu for clenched jaws; CV22 Tiantu and S40 Fenglong for gurgling with sputum; GV15 Yamen, L7 Lieque and H5 Tongli for aphasia and stiffness of the tongue.

Method: All the main points are prescribed with the corresponding auxiliary points according to the symptoms and the puncture is moderate. The needles are retained for 15 minutes and the treatment is given once daily.

B. The flaccid syndrome. The manifestations are coma, relaxed hands, agape mouth, closed eyes, pallor, profuse drops of sweat over head and face, and snoring. There may also be incontinence of feces and urine, cold limbs and feeble pulse. The prescription for puncture is:

Points: LI11 Quchi, CV4 Guanyuan and CV8 Shanque.

Method: All the above points are punctured with moderate stimulation. The needles are retained for 20 minutes and the therapy is given once daily.

The mild type. In this type, only the channels and collaterals are attacked and the symptoms pertain only to the channels and collaterals. The symptoms and signs are mostly those of the sequelae of the severe type, which involve the channels and collaterals. There are also primary cases without affliction of Zang-fu organs. Manifestations are hemiplegia or deviation of mouth due to motor or sensory impairment.

For hemiplegia. This again may be severe or mild and the attack may be on either side of the body. At the beginning, the affected limbs may be limp and later they become stiff, which finally leads to motor impairment. There may be dizziness and dysphasia.

Main points: GV20 Baihui, GV16 Fengfu and B7 Tongtian.

Auxiliary points: LI15 Jianyu, LI11 Quchi, TE5 Waiguan and LI4 Hegu for upper extremities; G30 Huantiao, G24 Yanglingquan and S36 Zusanli for lower extremities.

Method: All the main points are prescribed with the corresponding auxiliary points according to the symptoms. The needles are retained for 20 minutes and the therapy is given once daily.

*1. Herb therapy*

A. When the patient complains of disorientation, coughing with rales, coma, chest distress, with whitish glossy coating of the tongue and slippery pulse, the following formula is given.

Dao Tan Tang Jia Jian.

Constituents:

Dried old orange peel   12g
Pinellia   10g
Tuckahoe   10g
Licorice root   6g
Jack-in-the-pulpit   10g
Fruit of immature ciron or trifoliate orange   10g
Bulb of fritillary   10g
Tabasheer   10g
Root of purple-flowered peucedanum   15g
Apricot kernel   12g
Root of the narrow-leaved polygala   12g
Grass-leaved sweetflag   12g

Decoction and dosage. All the above herbs make a dose and six to ten doses are prescribed with one dose daily. Each dose is simmered twice and then the broth of each mixed, half of the mixed broth each time, twice a day.

B. When the patient has muscular atrophy and debility of the lower limbs with impaired mobility of the knees and ankle joints, which are caused by empty blood vessels, malnutrition of the muscles of the lower limbs, sensory disturbance of the skin, the following formula is prescribed.

Bu Yang Huan Wu Tang Jia Jian.

Constituents:

Milk veteh   40g
Chinese angelica   30g
Unpeeled root of herbaceous peony   30g
Chuanxiong   20g
Earth-worm   15g
Peach kernel   12g
Safflower   12g
Cassia   12g
Ox-knee   15g
Scorpion   10 pieces
Root of red rooted salcia   30g
Licorice root   6g

Decoction and dosage is the same.

In addition, injections prepared from the root of red rooted salvia and chanxiong are also very effective. 40cc of red rooted salvia injection plus 250 to 500cc of 10% glucose can be given intravenously once daily and a course lasts two weeks. Chuanxiong injection can be given alone intramuscularly, 80mg each time, or together with 500cc of 4% glucose once daily intravenously.

*3. Prophylactic measures*

Senile patients with deficiency of Qi and excessive sputum or with manifestations of hyperactivity of liver Yang such as dizziness and palpitation may sometimes present symptoms of stiffness of tongue, slurred speech and numbness of finger tips. There are prodromal signs of windstroke. Prophylactic measures are emphasizing diet and daily activities, avoiding over-straining. Frequent moxibustion on S36 Zusanli and B39 Xuanzhong may prevent the attacks.

# Chapter XIV
# INFECTIOUS DISEASES

## 1. PERTUSSIS (Whooping cough)

### GENERAL CONSIDERATION

The disease persists in unimmunized populations of the world as a highly contagious and potentially fatal disease of infants. It is caused by Bordetella pertussis (Hemophilus pertussis), first described by Bordet and Gengou in 1906. The illness is characterized by a catarrhal period of nonspecific respiratory symptoms that progresses to a stage of paroxysmal cough accompanied by the typical inspiratory whoop and vomiting. It may be complicated by potentially serious involvement of lower respiratory tract and the CNS. Protection from severe clinical infection usually follow an attack of pertussis.

In traditional Chinese medicine, the disease is called "Dun Ke," "Ji ke" and "Lu Ci Ke," which all mean an infectious disease frequently seen in children, caused by seasonal pathogens with obstruction of the air passages by putrid phlegm, and characterized clinically by chronic paroxysmal spasmodic coughs.

### CLINICAL MANIFESTATIONS

It is customary to divide the clinical course of whooping cough into three stages —catarrhal, paroxysmal and convalescent.

Catarrhal stage.

The catarrhal stage lasts for about 1 to 2 weeks. It begins with the symptoms of an upper respiratory tract infection or common cold, such as coryza, sneezing, lacrimation, cough, and low-grade fever. The child may appear listless and irritable. In the absence of a history of contact, whooping cough is not suspected. Sometimes the only manifestation is a dry hacking cough that excites little attention. After about a week the cough, instead of improving, gradually becomes more severe. It is likely to be especially troublesome at night and it begins to occur in paroxysms.

Paroxysmal stage.

The paroxysmal stage lasts, as a rule, 4 to 6 weeks, with outside limits of 1 to 10 weeks. The cough now comes in explosive bursts. A series of five to ten or more short, rapid coughs is given on one expiration and is followed by a sudden inspiration associated with a characteristic high-pitched crowing sound or whoop. During the attack, the child's face becomes red or cyanotic, the eyes bulge, the tongue protrudes, and the whole expression is anxious or utterly miserable. A number of paroxysms may be grouped together until, with the last one, the child succeeds in dislodging the mucous plug and brings up thick, tenacious material. Vomiting frequently follows the attack. Then the child often appears listless, dazed, or out of touch for a few minutes. The patient is likely to sweat profusely and to show facial edema, particularly around the eyes.

The number of paroxysmal attacks varies from four or five daily in mild cases to as many as 40 in more severe forms. The attacks are likely to occur more frequently at night than during the day time and more frequent in a stuffy room than in one well aired or outdoors. They may be precipitated by eating or drinking, by pressure on the trachea, by physical exertion, or by suggestion. Attacks tend to diminish during periods when the child's attention is concentrated on toys, puzzles, or books. Between attacks the patient is usually comfortable and does not seem ill. In some instances the typical whoop is not heard in spite of the severity and frequency of paroxysms. This is particularly true of infants under 6 months of age. In older persons and in those partially protected by vaccine, a typical mild attacks may occur in which only one or two whoops or none at all occur.

During the first 1 or 2 weeks of the paroxysmal stage, the attacks increase in severity and frequency. They remain at about the same level for a variable period, usually 1 to 3 weeks, and then gradually decline until the whooping and vomiting stop altogether.

Convalescent stage.

The convalescent stage is marked by cessation of whooping and vomiting. The number and severity of paroxysms decrease gradually. The cough usually lingers for a while, but its character is that of ordinary tracheitis or bronchitis; it fades away in about 2 or 3 weeks, with subsequent respiratory tract infections. Some patients will develop recurrent paroxysmal coughing attacks, complete with whoop and vomiting. These episodes may occur repeatedly for months or even for 1 or 2 years.

## DIAGNOSIS

Having once watched a typical paroxysmal attack and heard the whoop, the physician has little trouble in recognizing subsequent cases. The bursts of short, rapid coughs on one expiration followed by the high-pitched inspiratory crow and the hallmarks of no other disease. Even in the absence of the typical whoop, as in infants, the clinical diagnosis is strongly suggested by the paroxysmal nature of the cough. The red or cyanotic appearance and the associated vomiting.

During the catarrhal stage it is usually impossible to differentiate pertussis on clinical grounds from the common cold, bronchitis, or acute respiratory tract disease caused by various agents. A history of contact with a known case or a cough that becomes aggravated after a week should cause suspicion. It is important at this time to attempt to establish the diagnosis by isolation of B. pertussis from the nasopharynx.

The application of the fluorescent antibody technique to the diagnosis of pertussis offers a rapid method of identifying the organism after it has been isolated. However, it is not sufficiently specific to be used for examination of mucus or organisms from the throat.

The white blood cell count may contribute to the diagnosis. High counts with a predominance of lymphocytes are characteristic of whooping cough. At the end of the catarrhal phase, white blood cell counts of 20,000 to 30,000 per cubic millimeter, with 60 or more lymphocytes, are suggestive of the disease.

## TREATMENT

### I. Treatment in Western medicine.

#### 1. Specific treatment

Available evidence suggests that pertussis immune globulin may exert a beneficial effect on infants with severe disease. Pertussis immune serum globulin has been available for the treatment of pertussis since the mid-1940s. Physicians and "pertussis nurses" at that time believed that use of this preparation was followed by a decreased severity of paroxysms and vomiting and that the treated infants improved more quickly. Subsequent controlled studies did not confirm these impressions, since this question has never been fully resolved and since there are no ill effects caused by this preparation. The decision to use it should be made by the responsible physician, after assessing the individual patient.

The use of vaccines after onset of symptoms has not been shown to be effective and is not recommended.

Various antimicrobial agents have been used in conjunction with pertussis immune globulin, as well as independently. None has been established as effective in modifying the severity or shortening the course of the disease. Nevertheless, an antibacterial effect on B. pertussis has been shown in vitro from sulfadiazin and from broad-spectrum agents, including the tetracyclines, ampicillin, chloramphenicol, streptomycin and erythromycin.

#### 2. General treamtnet

Most cases are mild and the patient can usually be cared for at home.

Rest in bed is indicated as long as fever is present.

It is important to maintain proper nutrition with an adequate diet.

The use of moist oxygen and anticonvulsants is important for infants with respiratory complications manifested by dyspnea with or without cyanosis. The use of oxygen is also indicated for infants with convulsions.

Choking attacks caused by the accumulation of secretions in the pharynx must be promptly relieved by gentle aspiration with a soft catheter, repeated aspiration at intervals is useful in the prevention of such attacks. Close nursing supervision and timely aspiration may spell the difference between life and death.

### II. Treatment in traditional Chinese medicine.

#### Herb therapy

The paroxysmal stage. Cough is in explosive bursts and followed by a sudden inspiration associated with a characteristic high-pitched crowing sound or whoop, red tongue with little coating, rapid and small pulse. The general rule of treatment in traditional Chinese medicine is to enrich and moisten the lungs with sweet and cold drugs. The most commonly used formulas are:

Sang Xin Tang Jia Jian.

Constituents:

White mulberry leaf   10g
Apricot kernel  12g
Root of straight ladybell  10g
Bulb of fritillary  10g
Tasteless preserved soybean  10g
Capejasmine   10g
Tatarian aster   15g
Stemona  10g
Seed of pepperweed or flixweed tansymustard  15g
Congangrass rhizome  30g
Common reed rhizome  30g

Decoction and dosage. All the above herbs are put together into a boiler to be simmered twice and then the broth of each mixed, half of the mixed broth each time, twice a day. Two to four doses are prescribed.

Tao Hua San.

Constituents:

Twndril-leaved fritillary bulb  30g
Prepared gypsum   30g
Pinellia  12g
Musk  10g
Peppermint  10g
Borneol  6g
Cinnabar  6g

Preparation and dosage. Put all the herbs together and grind into fine powder. For 1-year-old children, 0.02g each time, three times a day. The increase of one year of age adds 0.01 to the dosage of each time and the total dose is no more than 0.3g.

The convalescent stage. Whooping and vomiting is markedly relieved, but the patient still complains of dry cough, afternoon fever, night sweat, malar flush, hot palms and soles, dry throat and hoarse voice, red and dry tongue, faint and rapid pulse. The treatment is to nourish the Yin and moisten the lungs with Yang Yin Qing Fei Tang Jia Jian.

Constituents:

Root of straight ladybell  15g
Tuber of dwarf lilyturf  20g
Root-bark of white mulberry  20g
Root-bark of Chinese walfberry  30g
Apricot kernel  15g

Snakegourd fruit  18g
Root of balloonflower  12g
Licorice root  6g
Fresh or dried root of rehmannia  20g
Root of Zhejiang figwort  20g
Bulb of fritillary  10g
Root of herbaceous peony  30g

Decoction and dosage is the same.

## 2. MUMPS (Epidemic parotitis)

### GENERAL CONSIDERATION

Mumps is an acute contagious disease caused by a paramyxovirus that has a predilection for glandular and nervous tissue. Mumps is characterized most commonly by enlargement of the salivary glands, particularly the parotid glands. One or more of the following manifestations of mumps may be associated with or may occur without parotitis: meningoencephalitis, orchitis, pancreatitis, and other glandular involvement. Inapparent infection occurs in a significant percentage of persons (30 to 40).

The disease is called "swollen cheek" in traditional Chinese medicine, and is thought to be caused by warm-heat pathogens. The cardinal clinical manifestations are swelling of the one or both parotid glands which are indistinctly outlined, elastic to palpation, painful and tender, and may be accompanied by fever and general malaise.

In traditional Chinese medicine, the condition is thought to be caused by certain seasonal wind or warm pathogens. Clinically, it is characterized by swelling of one or both parotid glands which are indistinctly outlined, elastic to palpitation, painful and tender, and may be accompanied by fever and general malaise, rapid pulse and yellow coating of the tongue.

### CLINICAL MANIFESTATIONS

For a long time the terms, mumps and epidemic parotitis, were used interchangeably. Mumps was recognized as primarily an infection of the salivary glands. The isolation of the virus and the development of the specific diagnostic and immunologic tests, however, have contributed to a better understanding of the pathogensis and a clarification of the clinical picture of the disease.

Infection with mumps virus usually develops after an incubation period of 16 to 18 days. In approximately 30% to 40% of the patients the resulting infection is inapparent. The remaining 60% to 70% of the patients develop an illness of variable severity with symptoms that depend on the site or sites of infection. In the majority of instances, clinical mumps is characterized only by parotitis, either unilateral or bilateral. Additional relatively common manifestations include submaxillary and sublingual gland infection, orchitis and meningoencephalitis. Pancreatitis, oophoritis, thyroiditis and other glandular infections are relatively rare. These various manifestations of mumps may precede, accompany, follow or occur without parotitis.

## DIAGNOSIS

The following factors should be pointed out as a diagnostic possibility:

A. A history of exposure to mumps 2 or 3 weeks before onset of the illness.

B. A compatible clinical picture of parotitis or other glandular involvement.

C. Signs of aseptic meningitis.

In the classic case of so-called epidemic parotitis, confirmatory laboratory procedures are usually unnecessary. In the absence of parotitis or in the presence of recurrent parotitis, however, the specific diagnostic aids whose description followed may have to be utilized.

Isolation of causative agent. Mumps virus can be recovered from the saliva, mouth washings, or urine during the acute phase of parotitis and from the CSF early in the course of meningoencephalitis. The isolation may be made by inoculating the amniotic cavities of 8-day-old chick embryos or susceptible cell cultures. The isolation of mumps virus is not a routine laboratory procedure.

Serologic tests. There are at least three serologic tests that are used to demonstrate the development of specific mumps antibody: complement fixation, hemagglutination—inhibition (HI), and virus neutralization. The CF test is the most practical and most reliable of these diagnostic procedures. The neutralizing antibody test is a more reliable indicator of susceptibility or immunity than the CF or HI antibody test.

The antibody becomes detectable in the blood by the end of the first week and the end of the second week a fourfold or greater rise in antibody titer can be demonstrated. When a diagnosis of mumps is suspected, acute and convalescent sera should be tested simultaneously. A fourfold or greater rise in the level of antibody confirms the diagnosis. This test is particularly useful for the diagnosis of mumps meningoencephalitis without parotitis.

## TREATMENT

### I. Treatment in Western medicine.

Mumps is a self-limited infection. The course of which is not altered by use of any of the antimicrobial drugs. Treatment is symptomatic and supportive measures are used. Aspirin or codeine will usually control the pain caused by glandular swelling. Warm applications seem to help some patients; others prefer cold. Topical ointments are useless. Parenteral administration of fluids is indicated for the support of patients with persistent vomiting associated with pancreatitis or meningoencephalitis.

### II. Treatment in traditional Chinese medicine.

*1. Herb therapy*

The most effective formula is Pu Ji Xiao Du Yin Jia Jian.

Constituents:

Skullcap   15g
Chinese goldthread   12g
Root of Zhejiang figwort   30g
Weeping forsythias   30g
Honeysuckle flower   30g
Dyers woad root   30g
Puff-ball   12g
Achene of great burdock   12g
Larva of a silkworm with batrytis   12g
Peppermint   12g
Chinese thorowax   30g
Skunk bugbane   12g
Root of balloonflower   12g
Gypsum   30g

Decoction and dosage. All the above herbs are put together into a boiler to be simmered twice and then the broth of each mixed, half of the mixed broth each time, twice a day. Two to four doses are prescribed.

*2. Acupuncture therapy*

Main points: S6 Jiache and LI4 Hegu.

Auxiliary points: LI11 Quchi for fever; Liv8 Ququan, Sp6 Sanyinjiao and Liv3 Taichong for the involvement of the testis and ovaries; L11 Shaoshang picked for severe pain.

Method: The main points are punctured before the auxiliary ones with either moderate or strong stimulation. The needles are retained for 20 to 30 minutes and the therapy is given once daily.

*3. Ear-acupuncture therapy*

Points: Parotid Pt, Cheek Pt, Sympathetic Nerve Pt and Shenmen Pt.

Method: Puncture all the points perpendicularly with strong stimulation. The needles are retained for 20 to 30 minutes with intermittent manipulation. The therapy is given once daily.

*4. Plum-blossom-needle therapy*

The areas for stimulation: the local swelling region and the area 1 cun lateral to the cervical column from the first to the seventh cervical vertebrae on both sides.

Method: The skin of the region is carefully sterilized and pecking goes in vertical lines from the upper to the lower part. Each line is pecked 5 times. The treatment is given once daily.

*5. Application therapy*

Fresh leaves of rumex madaio makino is smashed and applied on the swelling of the mumps.

**外国人学中西医结合疗法**

张俊文　白永权　等编著

\*

外文出版社出版

（中国北京百万庄路 24 号）

邮政编码 100037

北京外文印刷厂印刷

中国国际图书贸易总公司发行

（中国北京车公庄西路 35 号）

北京邮政信箱第 399 号　邮政编码 100044

1993 年（16 开）第一版

（英）

ISBN 7−119−01492− 7 / R・86（外）

03500

14−E−2733S